The **Vaccine** Book

The Vaccine Book

Making the Right Decision for Your Child

Robert W. Sears, M.D., F.A.A.P.

Little, Brown and Company
New York Boston London

Little, Brown and Company
Hachette Book Group
237 Park Avenue, New York, NY 10017
www.HachetteBookGroup.com

First Edition: October 2007

Little, Brown and Company is a division of Hachette Book Group, Inc. The Little,
Brown name and logo are trademarks of Hachette Book Group, Inc.

The information in this book is not intended to replace the medical care
or advice you receive from your doctor. You are encouraged to consult your
health care professional regarding the care of your child, and follow
his or her advice in the event of any conflict with any information contained
in this book. This book was written in July 2007, and the information
is correct as of this date. As new information becomes available through
research and experience, some of the data in this book may become invalid.
You are encouraged to seek the most up-to-date information on
medical care and treatment from your doctor or health care professional.

Library of Congress Cataloging-in-Publication Data

Sears, Robert, M.D.
The vaccine book : making the right decision for your child /
Robert W. Sears. — 1st ed.
p.   cm.
Includes index.
ISBN-10: 0-316-01750-7
ISBN-13: 978-0-316-01750-3
1. Vaccination of children.   2. Immunization of children.   I. Title.
RJ240.S42 2007
614.4'7083—dc22   2007022994

10   9

RRD-IN

Printed in the United States of America

To Gregg,
a dear friend and rocket scientist
who one day asked me a question
that really made me think . . .

Contents

VISIT DR. BOB SEARS ONLINE AT

WWW.THEVACCINEBOOK.COM

Vaccine information and research are constantly changing. New vaccines come into play, and older vaccines are sometimes taken off the market. New problems are found, and old problems are solved. I created TheVaccineBook.com to give you the most up-to-date information on vaccines and to offer you the resources that will help keep you informed. Here's what you will find:

- Vaccine topics in the news
- Disease outbreaks and epidemics
- Opinions and editorials on emerging vaccine issues
- Resources on how to boost your child's immune system
- Frequently asked questions answered
- Online forums for parents to chat together about vaccines
- Dedicated e-mail address for health care practitioners to send me questions and comments
- Schedules of my upcoming appearances, lectures, and conferences on vaccines
- How to order signed copies of *The Vaccine Book*
- How to find a doctor nearby who is open to discussing vaccines with you

Preface

Should you vaccinate your child?

This seems to be the question of the decade for many parents. It used to be "How can I get my baby to sleep through the night?" or "How can I get my toddler to eat better?" but today almost all parents have concerns about vaccines. In the old days, most parents simply followed their doctor's advice and automatically got their children vaccinated. But now virtually every parent has heard that there may be some side effects and other problems with vaccines, and they are confused. Their doctor tells them that vaccines are perfectly safe and they have nothing to worry about, but their friends tell them vaccines can be deadly and they are crazy to vaccinate. Faced with conflicting information, they have many questions. They don't want their child to catch any serious illnesses, but they want to know the potential risks and side effects of vaccines.

That's what this book is all about. It is my goal to give you a balanced look at the pros and cons of vaccination so that you can make an educated decision.

Before I tell you what I'm going to share with you in this book, allow me to first tell you what I'm *not* going to tell you:

I am not going to discuss at length mercury or thimerosal, be-cause, fortunately, these have been taken out of virtually all vac-cines. I will tell you which shots still have very small traces of mercury (about 1 percent of the amount that used to be there) and alert you to the few shots that still contain a full dose of mer-cury, but I'm not going to discuss how bad mercury is (or was). This issue is tragic for those families who feel their child was af-fected by mercury, but for those of you who are making the deci-sion today, mercury needn't be part of the equation. If you use the right vaccine brands and know in which vaccines mercury is still present, you can get the complete vaccine series 100 percent mercury free. On page 207 I'll give you all the pertinent facts you need to know about mercury.

I am not going to discuss the lengthy history of infectious dis-eases and vaccine discovery and evolution over this past century. While this is an interesting topic, I think it's information overload for the purpose of this book.

I am not going to discuss every last conspiracy theory and pos-sible shred of evidence suggesting that vaccines are harmful. We all know that vaccines have possible side effects. Just read any product insert; some of these side effects are potentially fatal. But, fortunately, they are extremely rare.

I want to be very clear on something right up front. This is not an *anti*-vaccine book. There are plenty of books out there that overemphasize the potential dangers of vaccines and leave par-ents even more fearful and confused.

So, enough about what this book isn't. Let's find out what it is. As I see it, vaccination isn't an all-or-nothing decision. There are many choices that can be made. Some parents choose all the shots, others choose only some vaccines, and a few parents choose no vaccines.

This freedom of choice, however, isn't enjoyed equally by all Americans. Our nation's public health service utilizes the public school registration process to verify that all children's vaccinations are up-to-date. Only twenty states allow parents to decline some or all vaccines at public school registration on the basis of personal beliefs. Twenty-eight other states allow parents to waive vaccines for school entry only if their religion dictates they do so. Since most religions have no problem with vaccines, this loophole isn't available to most people. Two states have mandatory vaccination laws. Parents who decline vaccination in these states can have their children taken away from them. I don't know if the authorities have ever gone this far in those two states, but the law does allow them to. Private schools, childcare centers, camps, and other recreational clubs in most states can set their own vaccine requirements. Some are more lenient and allow unvaccinated children into their programs. Even if you live in a state with strict requirements, you still have the freedom to choose which vaccines your baby will receive in the early years, before entering school. On page 217 I will give you more details on the various state requirements.

If you choose to have your child vaccinated, this book will answer your questions about how to proceed in the safest manner possible. Should she get all the shots together as they are recommended, or should you space them out a little bit? Are there one or two shots you might delay for now or skip altogether? Since there are currently twelve vaccines that are part of the routine childhood immunization schedule, parents have twelve separate decisions to make. If you thought you were going to have to make only *one* decision and I've just made your life a dozen times more complicated, I apologize. But when you have finished reading this book, you will have more answers than questions, and enough answers to make an educated decision for your child.

To keep things simple, each chapter discusses one vaccine/disease pair. I tell you what each disease is, how common it is, and how serious it is. I next tell you how the vaccine is made, what the ingredients are, and what the possible side effects are (not the imagined theoretical side effects, but the proven or highly suspected side effects). I then discuss the various points parents might consider when deciding if that vaccine is important for their child. I also share with you the steps you can take to minimize side effects when you do vaccinate your child. At the end of each chapter, I give my own brief summary about each vaccine. I don't ever tell you, "You must absolutely get this shot!" and I don't ever say, "You're crazy to give this vaccine to your child!" But I do offer you some insight about the relative importance of each shot. I also share my professional experience (if any) with each disease.

Are all vaccines equally important? No. You will learn that some diseases are more common and/or more deadly. Obviously, vaccines to prevent those diseases are more important, both for your child and from a public health standpoint. But a shot to prevent a disease that is extremely rare and usually harmless might be considered less important by some people. That's not to say that such a vaccine is unnecessary, because if such diseases run rampant throughout our nation, there will be some fatalities. Vaccine opponents claim the harm from the less important vaccines is worse than the occasional death from a disease. Most anti-vaccine books claim that all shots are bad, the diseases aren't really anything to fear, and as long as you live a natural and healthy lifestyle, you don't have to worry. I think this is a very irresponsible approach to the vaccine issue. Vaccines are beneficial in ridding our population of both serious and nonserious diseases. But families do have the right in our country to take their chances without vaccines.

Some people automatically think any book about vaccines is an anti-vaccine book. They assume the book is all about the dangers of vaccines and they dismiss it without even picking it up. I have actually been advised by some of my colleagues *not* to write this book because of the risk of this misconception.

I wrote this book because . . . *there is no other fully informed, unbiased vaccine book available.* Outside their doctor's office, parents have nothing to read that doesn't scare them away from vaccines. I don't want to leave you in the hands of the anti-vaccine books. I want you to know everything scientific there is to know about vaccines and the diseases they prevent. Because I've taken all my information from the vaccine product inserts and from medical journals and textbooks, you are getting the full picture your own pediatrician would probably give you if he or she had several hours to spend with you and had all this information memorized.

Some people feel that vaccine books aren't necessary; after all, why not just ask your doctor if vaccines are absolutely necessary and safe and leave it at that? It takes all of one minute, then you're done. No research or effort on your part is needed. Here's the problem with that approach. Doctors, myself included, learn a lot about diseases in medical school, but we learn very little about vaccines, other than the fact that the FDA and pharmaceutical companies do extensive research on vaccines to make sure they are safe and effective. We don't review the research ourselves. We never learn what goes into making vaccines or how their safety is studied. We trust and take it for granted that the proper researchers are doing their jobs. So, when patients want a little more information about shots, all we can really say as doctors is that the diseases are bad and the shots are good. But we don't know enough to answer all of your detailed questions about vaccines. Nor do we have the time during a regular health checkup to thoroughly discuss and debate the pros and cons of vaccines. That's why I've written this book. I've done the research. I've spent the last thirteen years learning everything I could about vaccines and the diseases they are designed to prevent, and I've put it all together in one place so you can get all your questions answered.

There is little doubt that vaccines have played a useful role in eliminating some diseases from our population and limiting many others. Smallpox is a case in point. We stopped giving this vaccine in 1969 because vaccination had succeeded in wiping the disease out in our country. Polio is another example of a disease that is no longer in the United States because of widespread vaccination.

Even though vaccines are important, you as a parent are still entitled to know what you are giving your child. You have a responsibility (and a desire) to make informed health care decisions for your family. Until recently, vaccines were viewed as an automatic part of childhood. But today's parents are taking a more active role in making choices for their child's medical care. That's what this book is all about—information. Open, honest, complete, and accurate information that all parents can use. It's taken me thirteen years to complete my journey to understanding the world of vaccines, but I hope to guide you through it in just a few days. So grab some coffee and a snack, sit back and put your feet up, and let's explore the vaccination decisions (all twelve of them) together.

A Note to Fellow Physicians

I know that much of the information in this book won't be new to you. But I am also aware that we receive little information on vaccines, other than that they are safe and effective in preventing diseases. Our education is focused mainly on the diseases themselves. So, what do I hope you will gain from this book? In my discussions on how common or rare each disease is, you might find this information more up-to-date than what you learned. You might also find the discussions on how each vaccine is made quite interesting. (I know I did.) The side effects sections are important to review, too. And you might learn something new about why some parents choose not to get a particular vaccine for their child. Finally, some of the last chapters on vaccine safety research, side effects, and ingredients are sure to stimulate your thinking.

We have all met patients who question the necessity and safety of vaccines. How should we respond to these patients? Where I practice, in Southern California, a number of pediatricians have dismissed families from their practices because of their refusal to have their child vaccinated. I'm not sure where this hard line comes from, because it goes against how the American Academy of Pediatrics says we should approach patients who decline vaccines. In *The Red Book* 2006, there is a section that advises doctors on what to do when their patients choose not to have their child vaccinated. Here is a brief summary:

- A nonjudgmental approach is best. Listen carefully and respectfully to the parent's concerns.

- Inform the parents of the risks and benefits of each vaccine as well as the risks of each disease.

- For parents who are concerned about multiple vaccines at one visit, develop a schedule that spreads the vaccines out.

- Continued refusal to vaccinate after adequate discussion should be respected (unless the child is at significant risk of serious harm during an epidemic).

- In general, pediatricians should avoid dismissing patients from their practice solely because of refusal to vaccinate.

The way I see it, a family that doesn't vaccinate needs a good doctor more than ever. It is my hope that through this book I can make your job (and mine) easier by giving your patients a complete and balanced look at the pros (of which there are many) and the cons (of which there *are* some) of vaccination. I know you don't have hours to spend with your patients to educate them on these vaccines and diseases. Let this book do it for you. I'm sure your patients will still have some questions for you, but this book and its resources can help you be more prepared.

When I set out to write this book, one of my goals was to take a close look at many of the theoretical problems with vaccines and to find conclusive medical evidence that showed these worries to be unfounded. I discovered that most of the risks and controversies over vaccination have been well researched in the medical literature, and there is much scientific evidence to show that vaccines are safe and effective in preventing diseases. Throughout the book I review many of these studies, covering a wide range of topics. However, I also found some issues that I believe haven't received adequate attention by researchers, and I offer suggestions for what further research needs to be done.

After you read this book, I welcome your feedback. I have a dedicated e-mail address just for physicians at www.TheVaccine Book.com, where you can send me your thoughts. I will personally consider each and every e-mail. You can also offer your experience and opinions on my physicians' message board. I want to create an online community of doctors who both agree and disagree when it comes to vaccine controversies. I also encourage you to register your medical practice information on my Web site if you want to make yourself more accessible to prospective patients in your community who are looking for a doctor to help them understand their vaccine options. Working together, we can educate our patients and make our nation's vaccine schedule the safest it can be.

A Note to the Reader

The information regarding how each vaccine is made, its ingredients, and its side effects is taken directly from each vaccine's product insert (PI). In some cases, I used other sources for some side effects. I noticed that a few PIs had changed over the years since I first began reading them thirteen years ago. While I have used the most up-to-date PIs for this book, it is possible that PIs will continue to change over the next few years, so information I have taken from a PI this year may vary slightly five years from now.

I discuss many different vaccine brand names and manufacturers. The names of the different vaccine manufacturing companies may also change over the years as companies merge and split. I will try to keep these up-to-date as I write revisions of the book.

Most of my information on diseases comes from *The Red Book* on pediatric infectious diseases, the most commonly used text for pediatricians in the United States. I also used articles and Web databases where needed and have cited these in my "Resources."

American Academy of Pediatrics
2007 Recommended Vaccine Schedule

Birth   Hep B

1 month   Hep B

2 months   HIB, Pc, DTaP, Rotavirus, Polio

4 months   HIB, Pc, DTaP, Rotavirus, Polio

6 months   HIB, Pc, DTaP, Rotavirus, Hep B, Flu

1 year   MMR, Chickenpox, Hep A

15 months   HIB, Pc

18 months   DTaP, Polio, Hep A, Flu

2 years   Flu

3 years   Flu

4 years   Flu

5 years   DTaP, Polio, MMR, Flu, Chickenpox

12 years   Tdap, Meningococcal, HPV (3 doses,
               girls only)

The **Vaccine** Book

1

Haemophilus Influenzae Type B and the HIB Vaccine

WHAT IS HIB?

HIB is a bacterium (singular for bacteria) that can cause serious illnesses such as meningitis (infection of the lining of the brain), blood infections, bone infections, and pneumonia. It is transmitted like the common cold (through contact with an infected person's cough, mucus, or saliva). Fortunately, when a person is exposed to HIB, the bacteria usually remain in the nose, ears, or throat and simply cause minor cold symptoms. Only rarely do they invade farther into the body and cause one of the severe infections mentioned above. Symptoms of these serious infections vary according to the body part that is affected but generally include fever, lethargy, vomiting, and a poor appetite. HIB is diagnosed through a blood test or spinal tap, tests that aren't done until a person is sick enough to go to the doctor. Because most cases of HIB go undiagnosed, no one knows exactly what percentage of minor HIB cases turn serious. This infection does not give a person lifelong immunity. It can be caught more than once.

The HIB Vaccine
American Academy of Pediatrics
2007 Recommended Vaccine Schedule

Birth	Hep B
1 month	Hep B
2 months	**HIB,** Pc, DTaP, Rotavirus, Polio
4 months	**HIB,** Pc, DTaP, Rotavirus, Polio
6 months	**HIB,** Pc, DTaP, Rotavirus, Hep B, Flu
1 year	MMR, Chickenpox, Hep A
15 months	**HIB,** Pc
18 months	DTaP, Polio, Hep A, Flu
2 years	Flu
3 years	Flu
4 years	Flu
5 years	DTaP, Polio, MMR, Flu, Chickenpox
12 years	Tdap, Meningococcal, HPV (3 doses, girls only)

IS HIB COMMON?

No, but it used to be. Before the vaccine came into use in the mid-1980s, there were about 20,000 cases of serious HIB infections each year in the United States. Now we have only about 25 cases each year, almost all occurring in children under age five and most in the first two years. It is very rare beyond age three. HIB can also occur in the elderly. Minor HIB infections (like simple runny noses or coughs) may be more common than this, but they are not tested for or diagnosed because they don't require medical attention.

IS HIB SERIOUS?

Yes. HIB meningitis has about a 5 percent fatality rate, and in about 25 percent of cases, there is some residual brain damage (such as hearing loss, learning problems, or nerve injury). Blood, bone, and lung infections, though less serious, are still potentially fatal. What makes HIB particularly dangerous is that it is difficult to recognize in its early stages. Often a parent can't tell her child has it until he is sick enough to see a doctor. If the child looks seriously ill, the doctor will order invasive testing. After that, it takes one or two days for a lab even to identify HIB in a blood sample.

IS HIB TREATABLE?

Yes. Intravenous antibiotics are given for several days in the hospital. This usually prevents fatalities, but, as in the case of meningitis, some permanent damage can result, especially if the diagnosis and treatment are delayed. In general, when a child is severely ill with a fever in the hospital, IV antibiotics are started right away while the lab tries to identify the infection from blood samples, so treatment for severe HIB disease is usually started before the germ is even identified.

In case you are wondering what the difference is between HIB meningitis and other types of meningitis, I will now tell you. There are dozens of different bacteria, viruses, and fungi that can infect humans and cause meningitis. HIB is just one of these causes, and it almost exclusively affects infants and the elderly. Pc (which you will read about in chapter 2) is very similar to HIB. *Meningococcus* (chapter 11) is a bacterium that can also cause meningitis, and at any age. And there are many other germs that cause meningitis that we don't have vaccines for yet. So, a person can catch any of these other types of meningitis even when fully vaccinated. Viral meningitis happens to be the most common type, and no vaccine yet exists for that.

WHEN IS THE HIB VACCINE GIVEN?

The HIB vaccine is given at two months, four months, six months, and fifteen months. (These intervals may vary slightly.) The last dose can be given anytime between twelve and fifteen months. The PedVaxHIB brand doesn't need to be given at six months because it works a little faster than the other brands. No booster dose is given later in childhood because the disease is almost unheard of beyond age three. This vaccine has been in use since approximately 1985.

HOW IS THE HIB VACCINE MADE?

All companies that make the HIB vaccine start with the same process: The HIB bacteria (presumably originating from an in-

---

WHY SO MANY DOSES?

Why do we give so many doses of a vaccine? In most cases, each shot creates only partial immunity to the disease, and subsequent shots build on that immunity. Some shots, like those for measles, mumps, and rubella and chickenpox, don't require a whole series to create immunity. This is because they are live-virus vaccines, which work well with one initial dose and sometimes a booster years later. As a general rule for shots that come in a series, the first dose provides approximately 50 percent immunity, the second dose bumps it up to about 75 percent, and the third dose gives around 90 percent immunity. A few diseases require a fourth dose about a year after the third, and then another booster dose about four years later. These are necessary to keep immunity levels high enough to be effective.

---

fected person decades ago) are nurtured in a culture medium, also called a petri dish. Batches of bacteria are removed from the petri dish and broken up, and the sugars that form the outer coating of the bacteria are filtered out, collected, and purified. The remaining portions of the bacteria are discarded. The sugars are then put into the vaccine solution.

Here is where the process varies by manufacturer:

ActHIB (Sanofi Pasteur, formerly Aventis Pasteur). Uses an additional tetanus toxoid (a chemical produced by the tetanus bacterium, not the actual bacterium itself) and attaches this toxoid to the HIB sugars.

PedVaxHIB (Merck). Takes a bacterium called *Neisseria,* breaks it up, and collects some proteins from the outer covering of the bacteria. These proteins are then bonded to the HIB sugars.

HibTITER (Wyeth). Uses a toxoid from the diphtheria bacterium (just like the ActHIB product uses a tetanus toxoid) to bind with the HIB sugars. Wyeth stopped making the HibTITER brand last year, and right now it has no plans to resume production. I don't know the reasons for this, but I have included the information here in case those of you with older children who may have received this vaccine want to look back at their vaccine record and read the details.

Why is the tetanus, *Neisseria,* or diphtheria part needed? They help the body's immune system recognize the HIB sugars and create a better response to the vaccine. The extra germ parts do not create any significant immunity themselves.

WHAT INGREDIENTS ARE IN THE FINAL VACCINE SOLUTION?

The ActHIB brand contains:

- HIB sugar/tetanus toxoid complex
- Sugar water
- Saline solution (salt water)

The PedVaxHIB brand contains:

- HIB sugar/Neisseria protein complex
- Saline solution
- Aluminum—225 micrograms (This makes the vaccine work a little better.) A microgram is 1/1000 of a milligram. (You probably can't picture how much that is. Neither can I.)

The HibTITER brand contains:

- HIB sugar/diphtheria toxoid complex
- Saline solution

DIFFERENT TYPES OF VACCINES

There are four main types of vaccines. The first is called a "poly-saccharide conjugate vaccine." This type uses only the sugars from the bacteria and bonds (conjugates) them to portions of another germ. It does not contain the entire germ, so there is no way to become infected with the disease from this vaccine. A second type of vaccine is a "live-virus vaccine." This vaccine contains the whole, living virus. It can actually give a person the infection, although fortunately that rarely happens. A third vaccine type contains the whole germ, but it has been killed, so it can't infect you. The fourth type of vaccine is called a "recombinant vaccine." It is genetically engineered and doesn't contain any portion of the original germ, though it does have some manufactured proteins that match the germ's proteins. As we go through the book, I will tell you which type of vaccine each one is. HIB is a polysaccharide conjugate vaccine.

Are any of these ingredients controversial?

The only item that is a potential problem is the aluminum in the PedVaxHIB brand. Although research has not proven that the aluminum in vaccines is harmful, some studies indicate that when too many aluminum-containing vaccines are given at once, toxic effects can occur. See page 193 for more information.

WHAT ARE THE SIDE EFFECTS OF THE HIB VACCINE?

This vaccine has one of the safest side effect profiles. The standard reactions, which occur in about 5 percent of babies, include fever, fussiness, redness and swelling, etc. ("Et cetera? What do you mean, 'et cetera'?" you may be asking right now. You don't want to just hear "et cetera" when it comes to possible side effects your child may experience. That's like a doctor telling you, "Your medicine may cause some side effects, but don't worry about it." On page 180 I go into more detail about the standard side effects that apply to all vaccines.)

Fortunately the HIB vaccine causes few serious reactions. The only serious side effects that have been reported are:

- *Guillain-Barré syndrome.* This disorder causes severe muscle weakness and paralysis. See page 181 for more details.

- *Serious HIB infection.* In the vaccine trials, more babies who received the vaccine caught a serious HIB infection than those who didn't get the vaccine. However, these infants didn't get infected by the vaccine itself. Research shows that while the vaccine is beginning to work on the immune system, the immune system can't react to a natural HIB infection for a period of five days. An immunized infant is therefore susceptible to catching natural HIB for a few days while her immune system is "distracted" by the vaccine. This may have been a problem back when HIB disease was common, but now that HIB is rare, the chance that a baby would be exposed to HIB during the few susceptible days after vaccination is minuscule. See "Resources," page 263, for the details on three studies in *The Journal of Pediatrics* and *The New England Journal of Medicine* about this side effect.

SHOULD YOU GIVE YOUR BABY THE HIB VACCINE?

Even though I pose this question in each chapter, I'm not going to answer it for you. Instead, I am going to present the logical points from both sides so you can make an informed choice.

Now, in case you are wondering exactly how I would know the reasons some people choose not to get a vaccine, I'll tell you. Whenever I meet a parent who doesn't vaccinate (or only partially vaccinates) her child, I like to pick her brain a little to see how she thinks. I've written down many responses over the years, and I've recorded the thoughtful and logical ones in this section of each chapter. (I've purposely left out any of the really, shall we say, "interesting" ideas. Although the inclusion of such interesting comments would be sure to entertain and amuse you—like the one about germs not really causing infections; they're just a normal and harmless part of our everyday existence, so the shots aren't needed to prevent them—some of them might just confuse the heck out of you, and this book is all about *un*-confusion.)

Reasons to get this vaccine

Obviously meningitis and blood infections are very serious. There are many germs out there that cause these conditions, and HIB used to be the most common one. Although HIB is now extremely rare, continued vaccination keeps the disease out of our population and will help protect your baby from the rare chance he may catch this germ. This shot also has the safest side effect profile of all the vaccines, and the ingredients are very pure compared with those found in most other vaccines.

Reasons some people choose not to get this vaccine

Probably the main reason some parents choose to skip this vaccine is that severe cases of this disease are now extremely rare (about 25 cases per year in the United States in kids under five years of age). A breastfed baby who does not attend day care is at a particularly low risk of catching this illness.

TRAVEL

Most of the information I provide regarding each disease pertains to people living in the United States. So, if I tell you a certain disease is rare and your child is at low risk of catching that disease, I am assuming that you are not planning to go be a missionary in Africa. In the case of each disease and vaccine, I briefly discuss whether you should be worried about that disease if you travel. When I say "travel," I don't mean vacation travel. Staying in hotels or on cruise ships and doing the normal tourist sightseeing doesn't typically put you in contact with the local diseases. But if you are planning to visit or live with relatives around the world for an extended period, or if you plan to live with the locals in the jungle for several weeks at a time, then you should carefully investi-

Travel considerations

While this disease is rare in the United States, it is still common in most other countries, since very few countries use the HIB vaccine. In my opinion, vacation travel doesn't pose much risk, but if you are planning to live with the locals for a while anywhere else in the world, you should consider the HIB vaccine for your infant if he or she is not yet vaccinated.

Options to consider when getting this vaccine

If you wish to be very cautious, you might want your baby to get only one or two aluminum-containing vaccines at a time. (See chapter 19 for how to make sure you get only one at a time.) Also,

gate the incidence of diseases there and consider vaccination for your child if she isn't fully vaccinated. In general, you need to begin vaccinating about three months before you travel in order to get adequate protection from a vaccine series. You can obtain more information about specific diseases in other countries at www.cdc.gov/travel/diseases.htm.

What about airplane travel itself? Flying for several hours and breathing the recirculated air theoretically could be risky for an unvaccinated baby. But this risk is probably very small. I'm not sure anyone has specifically researched this, however. If you have decided not to vaccinate your baby, I wouldn't say flying is risky enough for you to change your mind. In fact, flying is generally considered okay for a newborn baby, who is too young to have had any shots yet.

you can try to make sure your baby gets an aluminum-free brand whenever possible.

You have the option of getting the HIB vaccine in combination with the DTaP and polio vaccines in one injection instead of as three separate shots. This mix is called Pentacel (made by Sanofi Pasteur). Pentacel has been used in Canada for many years and has recently been approved for use in the United States. See page 40 for more details on this vaccine.

You also have the option to get Comvax (Merck). It is a combination of the HIB (PedVaxHIB brand; see page 5) and hep B (Recombivax brand; see page 54) vaccines in one shot. The manufacturing, ingredients, and side effects are the same as for the individual shots. This combination shot decreases the overall exposure to aluminum to 225 micrograms. Administered separately, the same Merck brands of HIB and hep B contain 475 micrograms of aluminum.

Another option to decrease the number of injections is the Tri-HIBit vaccine (Sanofi Pasteur). If your doctor uses the Tripedia brand of the DTaP vaccine (see page 33) and the ActHIB brand of the HIB vaccine (see page 5), these two can be mixed into one syringe for the eighteen-month dose (the fourth dose in the series). They can't be combined for the first 3 doses. The overall ingredients are the same as in the separate injections, but the number of injections is decreased by one. Any baby will appreciate that.

See page 153 for further discussion on choosing combo shots.

THE WAY I SEE IT

HIB is a bad bug. Fortunately, it's also a rare bug, so rare that I haven't seen a single case in ten years. Ongoing use of this vaccine in our country helps keep it that way. The HIB vaccine is one of the very safest we have. The ingredients aren't too strange, and the known side effects are minimal. Since the disease is so rare, HIB isn't the most critical vaccine. But it's definitely high on the Top Ten list.

2

Pneumococcal Disease and the Pc Vaccine

WHAT IS *PNEUMOCOCCUS?*

Pneumococcus (Pc) is a bacterium (the proper name is *Streptococcus pneumoniae*) that causes a wide range of illnesses, from mild cold symptoms and ear infections to severe pneumonia, bloodstream infections, and meningitis. It is transmitted like the common cold. When the germ finds its way into a person, it usually is kept restricted to the nose, throat, and ears and causes cold symptoms, coughing, or ear pain. Occasionally it moves down into the lungs and causes symptoms of pneumonia (labored breathing, severe cough, and fever). Very rarely the germ invades farther into the body and causes a bloodstream infection (symptoms include high fever and lethargy) or meningitis (fever, severe headache, vomiting, stiff neck). No one knows what percentage of the time Pc transforms from a minor illness into a more severe one, but this does happen more commonly in infants, toddlers, and the elderly.

Pneumococcal disease (Pc) is diagnosed with a blood test or spinal tap, but usually these are done only when a person is very

The Pneumococcal Vaccine
American Academy of Pediatrics
2007 Recommended Vaccine Schedule

Birth	Hep B
1 month	Hep B
2 months	HIB, **Pc,** DTaP, Rotavirus, Polio
4 months	HIB, **Pc,** DTaP, Rotavirus, Polio
6 months	HIB, **Pc,** DTaP, Rotavirus, Hep B, Flu
1 year	MMR, Chickenpox, Hep A
15 months	HIB, **Pc**
18 months	DTaP, Polio, Hep A, Flu
2 years	Flu
3 years	Flu
4 years	Flu
5 years	DTaP, Polio, MMR, Flu, Chickenpox
12 years	Tdap, Meningococcal, HPV (3 doses, girls only)

sick and a bloodstream infection or meningitis is suspected. Tests are not usually conducted to see if the germ that causes colds, ear infections, and pneumonia is actually *Pneumococcus.*

IS Pc COMMON?

Yes. It is a common bacterial cause of respiratory infections (although cold and flu viruses are still far more common). It is also the most common cause of infant meningitis. It has never been a reportable disease (one that automatically gets reported to the Centers for Disease Control by a lab or doctor whenever a case is detected), so we don't know exactly how common Pc is.

Since the vaccine came out in 2001, researchers have been gathering data on the number of cases of severe pneumococcal disease. One study showed that in kids under age five about 400 cases of severe Pc (meningitis, bloodstream infections, and pneumonia) have been reported each year by several major medical centers in large cities across the United States. Another report from a single large children's hospital in Dallas showed about 70 cases of severe Pc each year in that hospital alone. Hospitals across the country have reported 2000 to 3000 severe cases of antibiotic-resistant Pc each year in patients of all ages (these are just the severe cases in which the germ was found to be resistant to many antibiotics, not the total number of cases). The Centers for Disease Control estimate that there were about 60,000 cases of severe pneumococcal disease each year before the vaccine began. About 17,000 were in kids younger than five years of age. These numbers have seemed to decrease by at least half since the vaccine came into use, but now we are seeing increases in other strains of the Pc germ that are not covered by the vaccine. See "How Is the Pc Vaccine Made?" page 17, for more on this issue.

Overall, I estimate that there are about 10,000 cases of severe pneumococcal disease in young children each year, and another 20,000 to 30,000 in adults. Serious Pc infections (pneumonia, bloodstream infection, or meningitis) occur mostly in infants (ages two and under) and the elderly. Serious cases in healthy children and adults are uncommon.

IS Pc SERIOUS?

This depends on which body system is infected. Bloodstream infections have a 20 percent fatality rate (60 percent in elderly people), but those who survive usually don't have any lasting effects. Meningitis has a 30 percent fatality rate (80 percent in the elderly), and some of those who survive may have some brain damage or hearing loss. Pneumonia is fatal mainly in the elderly.

IS Pc TREATABLE?

Yes. Serious infections require hospitalization, with IV antibiotics for several days. Pneumonia can often be treated with oral antibiotics. Minor infections are treated with oral antibiotics.

WHEN IS THE Pc VACCINE GIVEN?

Currently one brand of Pc vaccine is widely used in the United States, called Prevnar (made by Wyeth). It is given at two months, four months, six months, and fifteen months to protect an infant for the first several years of life (when serious Pc is most likely to occur). The last dose can be given anytime between twelve and fifteen months of age. Although this vaccine usually isn't given after twenty-four months of age (the illness is very rare beyond that age), catch-up shots can be given through age five if any shots were missed.

There is a second brand of the Pc vaccine called Pneumovax 23 (made by Merck). It is an older version of the Pc vaccine that has never had widespread use in the general population. It is given only to people with certain immune disorders or chronic illnesses, who are highly susceptible to Pc disease, as well as to elderly people, who are prone to pneumonia. Only one dose is necessary for protection, with a booster three to five years later. It doesn't work well in infants and toddlers (this is why the new version was developed).

HOW IS THE Pc VACCINE MADE?

To make Prevnar, seven strains of Pc germs are kept alive in a soy culture. (The original source of the germs is unknown, but they probably came from infected patients many years ago.) As with the HIB vaccine, the bacteria are broken up and some sugars from the outer covering of the germs are filtered out and purified using several filtering techniques. Also, diphtheria bacteria are grown in a yeast culture. Toxins produced by the diphtheria bacteria are then extracted and purified into a toxoid (as in the HIB vaccine manufacturing process; see page 4). The Pc sugars and diphtheria toxoid components are then combined with aluminum. The diphtheria and aluminum help the vaccine work better. Since this isn't a whole-cell or live-virus vaccine, there is no way to become infected with Pc from this shot. The Pc vaccine is classified as a polysaccharide conjugate vaccine (see page 7).

When the Prevnar vaccine was first developed, the seven strains of the Pc bacteria used to make it were the seven most commonly found strains in our population. However, now that the vaccine has greatly reduced those seven strains in our population, others are emerging. A brand-new study (see "Resources," page 268) showed that 96 percent of the severe cases of Pc disease at Children's Medical Center in Dallas were caused by Pc strains not found in the vaccine. Researchers are already working on updated versions of the Pc vaccine in order to accommodate these emerging strains. I will provide updates as they develop at www.TheVaccineBook.com.

The Pneumovax 23 brand is made of sugars from the outer coating of twenty-three different strains of Pc in a saline solution with phenol as a preservative.

WHAT INGREDIENTS ARE IN THE FINAL VACCINE SOLUTION?

- Pc sugar/diphtheria toxoid complex
- Aluminum—125 micrograms

Are any of these ingredients controversial?

- The aluminum is the only controversial ingredient. See page 193 for a detailed discussion of the controversy of injected aluminum.

WHAT ARE THE SIDE EFFECTS OF THE Pc VACCINE?

The standard reactions (see page 180) occur in about 20 percent of babies, a higher frequency than from the HIB and DTaP vaccines.

In 2004 *The Journal of the American Medical Association* published data on the side effects of Prevnar (see "Resources," page 268). In the first two years of Prevnar's use in the United States, about 32 million doses were given, and about 4100 adverse reactions were reported to the Vaccine Adverse Events Reporting

System (see page 163 for more on VAERS). Most reactions were fairly mild, but about 15 percent (around 600) were considered serious. This means that for every 53,000 doses, one serious reaction occurred. Of course, we don't know that the reactions were caused by the vaccine, since some events occurred more than a month after the shot, and most infants were given several shots at once, not just Prevnar. See page 181 for a detailed discussion of serious vaccine reactions.

One particular side effect that stands out from this data is seizures. We know seizures can occur after any vaccine (usually due to high fever, not from the actual vaccine), but four hundred seizures were reported in babies over this two-year period. (Many of them already had a previous history of seizures.) That comes out to about a seizure for every 80,000 doses. Since each baby gets 4 doses, this means that about one in 20,000 infants may have a seizure after this vaccine. While this is a fairly rare occurrence, it seems to happen more commonly with Prevnar than with most other vaccines. Fortunately, most seizures were a one-time occurrence, not the beginning of a chronic seizure disorder.

There are many side effects listed in the product insert for the less common Pneumovax 23, but all are extremely rare.

SHOULD YOU GIVE YOUR BABY THE Pc VACCINE?

Reasons to get this vaccine

Most parents realize that Pc can be a very serious infection. It occurs mainly in infants and in the elderly, so it makes sense to immunize babies. Pc is fairly common now, but I hope that in ten years it will be as rare as HIB is now. The ingredients are comparatively safe, and the known side effect profile is fairly safe.

**BREASTFEEDING AND AVOIDING DAY CARE HELP
PROTECT A BABY FROM INFECTION**

As you read about the diseases in this book and consider your baby's risk of catching each one, keep this in mind: If your baby is breastfeeding, his chance of catching any of these illnesses is greatly reduced. Breast milk has antibodies that coat the lining of the nose, lungs, and intestines, so most germs that get inhaled or swallowed are killed.

When I see patients in the office who tell me they don't want their baby to get vaccines, my first response is, "I hope you plan to breastfeed your baby for at least two years!" If the parents answer, "Yes, of course we are," I breathe a sigh of relief. Breast milk passes a whole host of mom's antibodies for a variety of diseases to the baby. If they tell me, "Well, no. We just weaned our two-

---

Reasons some people choose not to get this vaccine

The main reason some choose not to get this vaccine is probably the higher-than-average rate of seizures and other standard side effects. Also, some parents worry that the more reactive a shot is, the greater the risk of permanent injury from that vaccine. Research hasn't shown this relationship, but some parents worry nonetheless. You can read more about vaccine reactivity on page 184.

Another reason some parents might decline this vaccine is that if their baby is breastfed and not in a large group day care, he has a lower-than-average risk of catching this disease.

month-old and are now using formula," I worry. Of course, even a breastfed baby can get sick. But the chance is lower.

When parents tell me they don't want their baby vaccinated, I like to assess their baby's overall risk. Placing a young baby in a group day-care setting significantly increases a baby's risk of encountering diseases, including meningitis, pertussis (whooping cough), rotavirus, measles, mumps, rubella, chickenpox, hepatitis A, and the flu. An unvaccinated baby in day care is very likely to catch at least one of these infections during his first few years.

Furthermore, if an unvaccinated baby is in day care *and* is not breastfed, he is really asking to get sick. Parents who choose not to vaccinate should avoid day care and should breastfeed for as long as possible. It would be prudent to even avoid church nurseries and health club childcare centers for the first year or two.

Travel considerations

Since this vaccine is a fairly recent addition to the U.S. schedule, the disease is still as common here as it is in the rest of the world. So right now international travel isn't any riskier than day-to-day life in the United States. Perhaps in ten years, when pneumococcal disease is dramatically reduced here, travel to countries where this vaccine isn't in use may pose an increased risk to unvaccinated Americans.

Options to consider when getting this vaccine

Since the Pc vaccine contains aluminum, babies should not get this shot in the same month as other aluminum-containing shots, if possible. Although research has not proven that the aluminum in vaccines is harmful, some research shows that when too much aluminum is given at once, some toxic effects can occur. If you are really curious about this and can't wait until the end of the book to read more on aluminum, skip to page 193 to satisfy your curiosity. Also, see chapter 19 for how to make sure you get only one aluminum-containing vaccine at a time.

THE WAY I SEE IT

Pc diseases can be very bad or only minor irritations. The problem is, you don't know until you're stuck with one. The Pc germ is a fairly common resident in day cares, schools, and checkout lines at the grocery store. Unless you are a housebound agoraphobic or a stay-at-home mom who never, ever takes her baby out, you and your kids *will* encounter this germ. The Pc vaccine offers a "get out of jail free" card, so to speak. The shot does come with some possible side effects, but fortunately these are rare. Overall, I'd call this a fairly important vaccine.

I've seen only one serious case of Pc infection in my office in my ten years of practice. A six-month-old unvaccinated baby had a Pc ear infection that spread to the skull bones behind the ear. She required surgery and IV antibiotics. Afterward, I asked parents if they regretted their decision to not vaccinate. They said no. They were both well-educated professionals, had done a lot of reading on this issue, and still felt comfortable with their decision.

3

Diphtheria, Tetanus, and Pertussis Diseases and the DTaP Vaccine

Diphtheria

WHAT IS DIPHTHERIA?

Diphtheria is a very severe throat infection that is caused by a bacterium (*Corynebacterium diphtheriae*). The germ secretes a toxin that irritates the lining of the throat and upper lungs, causing severe coughing and breathing difficulty. The breathing passage becomes swollen and may close off altogether. There isn't a reliable way for parents to be sure if their child has this specific infection. But the severe breathing difficulty would prompt any parent to seek urgent medical attention, at which time the diagnosis would be made by sending a cotton swab of the throat to a lab for testing. Diphtheria is transmitted like the common cold.

IS DIPHTHERIA COMMON?

No. Early in the twentieth century there were about 200,000 cases each year in the United States. In recent decades there have

The DTaP Vaccine
American Academy of Pediatrics
2007 Recommended Vaccine Schedule

Birth	Hep B
1 month	Hep B
2 months	HIB, Pc, **DTaP**, Rotavirus, Polio
4 months	HIB, Pc, **DTaP**, Rotavirus, Polio
6 months	HIB, Pc, **DTaP**, Rotavirus, Hep B, Flu
1 year	MMR, Chickenpox, Hep A
15 months	HIB, Pc
18 months	**DTaP**, Polio, Hep A, Flu
2 years	Flu
3 years	Flu
4 years	Flu
5 years	**DTaP**, Polio, MMR, Flu, Chickenpox
12 years	**Tdap**, Meningococcal, HPV (3 doses, girls only)

been a maximum of only 5 cases each year, and many years go by without any reported cases at all.

IS DIPHTHERIA SERIOUS?

Yes. About 10 percent of cases are fatal. Sometimes the germ and toxin have done so much damage by the time treatment is started that the victim dies.

IS DIPHTHERIA TREATABLE?

Yes. An antitoxin (a substance that neutralizes the germ's toxin) is given intravenously, and antibiotics are given to kill the germ.

(Here's an interesting historical note: The animated movie *Balto* is based on a true story of a diphtheria outbreak that threatened the isolated town of Nome, Alaska, in 1925. Sled dogs—Balto being the bravest!—had to travel 674 miles to bring the antitoxin to save the town. The Iditarod sled dog race is a commemoration of this event. There's even a statue of Balto in New York's Central Park. I've got pictures of my kids climbing on it!)

Tetanus

WHAT IS TETANUS?

Tetanus is an acute infectious disease that is caused by a bacterium that lives in soil and on dirty, rusty metal and can also contaminate unsterile needles. Once introduced into a deep, dirty wound or through a needle, the germs multiply and secrete a toxin that enters a person's nerves and gradually causes paralysis throughout the entire body. Tetanus is commonly referred to as lockjaw because often the first muscles to become paralyzed are the jaw muscles.

IS TETANUS COMMON?

No. Most people with deep and dirty wounds receive proper medical care and have their wounds flushed out with clean water and disinfectant. Each year in the United States we see only about 50 to 100 cases of tetanus. Virtually all occur in adults over twenty-five who haven't received a booster shot. Only about 1 case occurs in kids under five each year, and only a handful in older children. Before this vaccine was introduced several decades ago, about 1300 cases were reported each year in the United States.

Internationally, tetanus is a much more severe problem for infants. The World Health Organization reports that about two hundred thousand infants die each year from tetanus worldwide. This occurs most often when an unvaccinated mom gives birth, the umbilical cord is cut with a dirty tool, and tetanus spores from the dirty tool flow into the newborn baby through the cord. This doesn't happen in developed countries.

IS TETANUS SERIOUS?

Yes. It has a 15 percent fatality rate.

IS TETANUS TREATABLE?

Yes and no. Tetanus antibody injections and antibiotics can help eliminate the germs, but there is no medication that will reverse the paralyzing toxin. It just has to run its course. A person needs intensive care and life support while the paralysis wears off. This may take a few weeks.

If an unvaccinated person gets a deep puncture wound that can't easily be flushed out or a large, deep wound with dirt in it, a vaccine at that time may help prevent tetanus. It isn't as effective as already having the series of shots in your system, though. If the wound has a very high chance of causing tetanus, a tetanus antibody injection can also be given to an unvaccinated person. This tetanus immune globulin (TIG) can immediately inactivate any tetanus bacteria present. TIG is made from antibodies that are filtered out of donated human blood units and then treated and sterilized with various chemicals and filtering steps.

Pertussis

WHAT IS PERTUSSIS?

Otherwise known as whooping cough, pertussis is caused by a bacterium (*Bordetella pertussis*) that infects the upper lungs. It secretes a toxin that causes severe irritation and damage to the lining of the upper lungs and throat. Pertussis is similar to diphtheria, but not as serious. Symptoms mimic the common cold in the first week, but then the cough worsens into prolonged coughing fits that last from thirty seconds to as long as two minutes. The cough is so severe that a person can barely breathe, and when a breath is finally possible, it sounds like a gasping "whoop." Pertussis is transmitted like the common cold and can last for as long as three months, even with treatment. Infection usually creates lifelong immunity, but this natural immunity isn't perfect. To ensure immunity, the general medical recommendation is to continue with vaccination even after a person has had the disease.

Usually a doctor can diagnose pertussis just by hearing a description of the severe coughing spells or by observing such a spell. When the diagnosis is in doubt, a nasal swab inserted about three inches into the back of the nose, or saline squirted into the nose and suctioned out to collect mucus, can be sent to a lab. There are two ways to test for pertussis germs. One test takes about two days but it is only about 50 percent sensitive (it detects the germs only about half the time). Moreover, it tests positive only if done during the first few weeks of the illness. The other test is a culture, but the germ can take a week or two to show. Given the drawbacks of these tests, most doctors skip them and just treat for pertussis whenever it is suspected based on the coughing spells.

IS PERTUSSIS COMMON?

Yes. There were approximately 10,000 reported cases each year in the United States during the 1990s and early 2000s. This increased to about 25,000 reported cases in 2004 and again in 2005. Over the past few decades, pertussis has seemed to peak mysteriously every five years and then decline again. The 2004–2005 peak (which is the highest in many years) seems to be just another temporary rise, because in 2006 only 13,000 cases were reported. It looks like reported cases will reach only 10,000 in 2007. In the early part of the twentieth century, before the pertussis vaccine came out in the 1940s, there were about 240,000 cases each year in the United States.

What makes pertussis so common is that when teens and adults get infected, they don't necessarily have such severe coughing fits. Their coughs look more like a common bronchitis, so they tend to go longer without treatment and spread the disease around for several weeks. Since most adults lose their pertussis immunity (the childhood shots wear off), they are an endless breeding ground for this disease. For that reason, pertussis will probably never be eradicated from the world the way some other diseases have been. The number of reported cases each year are just those that are diagnosed. The actual number of cases is likely much higher when we take into account the undiagnosed adults.

IS PERTUSSIS SERIOUS?

Yes. Pertussis is most serious in the first six months of life, with about a 1 percent fatality rate for that age group. Recent studies show that of the approximately 2000 reported cases of pertussis each year for infants less than six months, about 75 percent are hospitalized and about twenty die each year. Most of these deaths occur before two months of age (see "Resources," page 267). The coughing fits can last so long that the infant is unable to breathe for a minute or so. This deprives the brain of oxygen and can cause brain damage. Fortunately, this is extremely rare—about 10 cases each year. There are almost never any long-term effects from this disease. The coughing slowly resolves and the lungs recover over a couple of months.

Beyond six months of age, fatalities from pertussis are almost unheard of, so it isn't considered a serious disease in older infants, children, and adults. We continue to vaccinate beyond infancy in order to decrease the disease in our population and protect infants. During the year that I wrote this book, seven infants less than two months of age died of pertussis in my state of California. They were too young to have even had the vaccine yet. This is an example of how older kids and adults can easily spread the disease to vulnerable babies.

IS PERTUSSIS TREATABLE?

Yes and no. Antibiotics are used to kill the germ, so a person is no longer contagious. However, the damage to the airway caused by the infection produces weeks of ongoing cough, even after the germs are gone. If treatment is started right at the onset of the coughing fits, the disease course may be milder and shorter. But by the time anyone realizes a bad cough is actually pertussis, treatment might not help very much and the disease will just need to run its course. Infants who have severe coughing fits and turn blue each time due to lack of oxygen need to be hospitalized for several days to help support them through the fits. A person is no longer considered contagious after five days of antibiotics.

WHEN IS THE DTaP VACCINE GIVEN?

Various types of D, T, and P vaccines have been used for many decades, but the current DTaP has been in use in the United States since the early 1990s.

DTaP is given at two months, four months, and six months to give babies protection during the time the disease is most dangerous. A booster is given at fifteen or eighteen months to provide protection through toddlerhood. Another booster is given at five years to add many more years of protection. This last dose can be administered anytime between four and six years.

REPORTED CASES OF DISEASES VERSUS ACTUAL CASES

Throughout this book I cite the number of cases reported annually for each disease. But this number isn't always the true number of cases. Diseases are diagnosed in one of two ways: Some are diagnosed just by observation by a doctor and some are diagnosed through blood testing. Diseases like pertussis, measles, mumps, rubella, chickenpox, hepatitis A, the flu, and rotavirus are often diagnosed by a doctor in the office but not actually tested for (although testing is available for all of these at the discretion of the doctor). If the doctor remembers to report it to the public health department, it gets counted as a confirmed case for the year. But this often doesn't happen. In addition, sometimes these diseases aren't even recognized and the patient recovers without ever getting diagnosed. It is estimated that the true number of cases of these diseases may be two to ten times the reported number.

On the other hand, diseases like hepatitis B, meningitis (HIB, pneumococcal, and meningococcal), and polio are diagnosed using actual tests, so even if a doctor forgets to report it, the laboratory almost definitely does. So, the reported numbers of these diseases are probably fairly accurate (except for cases that don't seek medical care, such as mild cases of hepatitis or Pc disease).

A new change in 2006 was the addition of a teenage booster dose of the DTaP vaccine. The main reason for this is that pertussis is common among teens and adults. While it isn't so serious for them, it does increase the spread of the illness to infants. This teen booster dose is recommended for kids age eleven or twelve (or anytime later if they missed it) and is called Tdap. Another new recommendation is that adults get the new Tdap vaccine every ten years (instead of just the tetanus booster, as has been done in past years). This will help decrease pertussis in the adult population, thereby decreasing the occurrence in infants. The vaccine is especially recommended for new moms right after the baby is born (it isn't approved during pregnancy yet). Dads can even get the vaccine while the mom is still pregnant. This decreases both parents' risk of catching pertussis and passing it along to their baby during the first two months of life when the disease is most serious and the baby can't yet be vaccinated himself.

HOW IS THE DTaP VACCINE MADE?

The diphtheria and tetanus components. These germs are grown in cultures, and the toxins produced by the germs are filtered out and purified using formaldehyde. The germs are discarded.

The pertussis component. The pertussis bacteria are grown and maintained in a culture. Batches of the germs are then broken apart, and various proteins and toxins from the germ are extracted using several filtering and purification techniques. Formaldehyde is added to make the germ components and toxins inactive in order to minimize adverse reactions.

The three components of the vaccine are then combined. Aluminum is added to increase the vaccine's effectiveness. Since this isn't a whole-cell or live-virus vaccine, there is no way to become infected with any of the diseases in this shot.

Two brands of DTaP vaccine (Infanrix and Tripedia) use cow tissue extract in their tetanus and/or diphtheria culture to nourish the germs. The other brand (Daptacel) does not use cow extract. Now, I'm not sure what cow extract is, but it's some sort of liquid made from cow parts. (See page 191 for a discussion of the implications of using animal tissues to make vaccines.) Another theoretical benefit of the Daptacel brand is that it contains less than half the quantity of pertussis components of the others. When it comes to vaccines you might think more is better, but that's not necessarily true. In this case, since it is the pertussis components that are thought to trigger most side effects, less may end up being better.

WHAT INGREDIENTS ARE IN THE FINAL VACCINE SOLUTION?

The Daptacel brand (Sanofi Pasteur) contains:

- Three germ and toxoid components (described above)
- Saline solution
- 2-phenoxyethanol (an alcohol solution used as a preservative)
- Aluminum—330 micrograms
- Formaldehyde—100 micrograms (Exactly how much is that? It makes up about 0.02 percent of the vaccine solution.)

The Tripedia brand (Sanofi Pasteur) contains:

- Three germ and toxoid components (described above)
- Saline solution
- Aluminum—170 micrograms
- Formaldehyde—100 micrograms
- Polysorbate 80—a preservative used in various vaccines
- Mercury—less than 0.3 micrograms

The Infanrix brand (GlaxoSmithKline) contains:

- Three germ and toxoid components (described above)
- Saline solution
- Aluminum—625 micrograms

- 2-phenoxyethanol
- Polysorbate 80—100 micrograms
- Formaldehyde—100 micrograms

What are all these strange chemicals? See page 207 for a discussion of the various chemicals used in vaccines.

ADOLESCENT AND ADULT Tdap

As you will notice, the *d* and the *p* in the name of the vaccine are both lowercase. This is because the vaccine contains less diphtheria and pertussis than DTaP does, since teens and adults react with more side effects when given the full dose of these components. There are two brands of this vaccine:

Boostrix (GlaxoSmithKline). In ingredients and manufacturing, it is similar to the infant DTaP vaccine made by GlaxoSmithKline (Infanrix), except that there is no 2-phenoxyethanol and less aluminum in Boostrix (only 390 micrograms).

Adacel (Sanofi Pasteur). In ingredients and manufacturing, it is almost identical to the infant DTaP made by Sanofi (Daptacel), except that there is much less formaldehyde in Adacel.

Are any of these ingredients controversial?

Compared with some vaccines, DTaP has a lot more chemicals in it:

- Aluminum. See page 193 for a discussion of the possible effects of this metal.
- Formaldehyde. This is a known toxic chemical. (Remember the frogs you dissected in your high school biology class? That smell

"I THOUGHT THERE WAS NO MERCURY IN VACCINES TODAY"

You may recall that in my preface I said you no longer have to worry about mercury and that mercury is no longer a big issue. Yet the Tripedia brand still has a bit of mercury, so what gives? Here's the deal: Tripedia used to have 25 micrograms of mercury in each dose. The manufacturer has tried to filter it all out, but the filter can't get every tiny last bit of it, so a residual amount is left over—about 1 percent of what used to be there. So, technically speaking, while this vaccine isn't mercury free, it sure is much safer than before. The tiny amount that remains is negligible. This is also true of a couple of other vaccines that I will point out later. You should be aware, however, that two vaccines still contain the full dose of mercury (as of late 2007)—two brands of the flu shot and the large multidose vials of the plain tetanus vaccine. I'll point these out to you when we get to them later in the book. See page 207 for a summary of vaccines that still have traces of mercury.

was formaldehyde, and you probably inhaled far more of it than is contained in a vaccine). See page 209 for more information on formaldehyde.

- Polysorbate 80 and 2-phenoxyethanol. Both are toxic in large amounts. The trace amount in the shot is probably harmless. See pages 209 and 210 for more information.

WHAT ARE THE SIDE EFFECTS OF THE DTaP VACCINE?

The *P* component of this vaccine has a bad reputation. That's because the older form of the shot (the whole-cell DTP vaccine, which had the entire pertussis germ in it) caused some very serious reactions (such as shock, seizures, and brain dysfunction). In the mid-1990s the most reactive components of the germ were removed (the *a* in DTaP stands for "acellular," meaning "containing no cells"), so now we see fewer, and less severe, side effects. The bad things you may have read about the DTP vaccine (and there are some very thoroughly researched books and articles on this topic) do not apply to the DTaP vaccine. See "Resources," page 265, for several articles that discuss the problems with the old DTP vaccine.

The standard side effects (see page 180) occur more often with the DTaP than they do with the HIB vaccine, but less often than with Prevnar. About 15 percent of babies have a standard side effect.

The serious reactions that have been reported with the DTaP vaccine are Guillain-Barré syndrome, brain damage, and other nerve dysfunctions. According to the Institute of Medicine (a very well-respected group of doctors and researchers) and the Daptacel and Adacel product inserts, there have been enough cases of Guillain-Barré syndrome (see page 181), nerve dysfunction (usually the nerves in the arm or face), and encephalopathy (possible permanent dysfunction of parts of the brain) to say that it is the tetanus toxoid component of vaccines that may cause these reactions. That makes sense, since in a real tetanus infection, it's the toxin that moves into the nerves and causes paralysis, and there is a modified tetanus toxin in the vaccine. Thankfully, these reactions are rare, although to my knowledge no one has calculated how rare.

Other reported reactions

Over the many years of use, the following have been reported with enough frequency to warrant making the list of possible reactions. In most cases, there have been twenty or more reports. We don't know out of how many doses such reactions occur, but it is somewhere in the realm of tens of millions, if not hundreds of millions. You could probably say your baby has a one in a million chance of having one of the following reactions:

- Pain and swelling of the lymph nodes
- Heart inflammation
- Extensive and serious swelling of the injected limb
- Diabetes
- Seizures
- Bruising throughout the body
- Bleeding disorders
- Blue color from poor circulation
- Severe allergic reactions
- Skin infections

Side effects of the adolescent and adult Tdap

The standard side effects occur more frequently (in about 25 percent of patients) with this shot than with the DTaP given to infants. Headache and fatigue were the most common (30 to 40 percent). The other side effects listed for DTaP have also been seen with Tdap.

SHOULD YOU GIVE YOUR BABY THE DTaP VACCINE?

Reasons to get this vaccine

Pertussis is a common disease, and it is most serious in the first six months of life. These are good reasons to follow the AAP guidelines and have your baby get this vaccine during infancy. Booster shots at eighteen months and five years are also a logical idea, since they decrease the spread of pertussis among school-age kids (and thus to their baby siblings). Vaccinating teens and adults who are around babies also makes good sense. Although pertussis was on the rise, it is declining again. But the less we vaccinate, the more common the disease will become, with more infant fatalities.

Diphtheria, while extremely rare in the United States, is a very dangerous disease. Vaccinating helps keep it out of our population. It's also a potential hazard during international travel (read on).

Tetanus, while not a disease of infancy, is serious when the very rare case does occur in a child. Giving the vaccine series while a person is young is a convenient way to make sure a child has tetanus protection while he grows up.

Reasons some people choose not to get this vaccine

In truth, tetanus is not an infant disease, and virtually all cases occur in adults. Also, diphtheria is virtually nonexistent in the United States. So, one could create a logical argument that a baby could skip the tetanus and diphtheria shots for a few years and be just fine. This child could then get the tetanus series as a teenager, and the diphtheria shots before traveling the world. He could even get them together as the DT shot.

The chemical components of this vaccine, more so than any other vaccine, are a concern to some parents. The negative press over the old DTP vaccine weighs heavily on the minds of some parents who worry that the newer vaccine may not be safe enough.

The cow tissue extract used in two of the brands may concern some parents (see page 191 for more on the issue of using animal and human tissues to make vaccines).

Now for the real quandary: Some parents may feel that their baby doesn't need tetanus and diphtheria protection just yet, but the high rate and potential severity of pertussis does concern most people with a new baby. They may want to get their baby vaccinated for pertussis only. The problem is, there is no pertussis-only vaccine. There is a tetanus-only vaccine, and there is a diphtheria-tetanus vaccine. But if a baby is going to get pertussis protection, he has to get the entire DTaP vaccine. So, skipping the DTaP because you don't think your baby needs D and T protection leaves him vulnerable to P, but giving the DTaP series for P protection also gives your baby vaccines for two diseases he is unlikely to get. Unfortunately, there is no way around this problem at present.

Travel considerations

To get the most up-to-date information on where these diseases are found in other parts of the world, visit www.cdc.gov/travel/diseases.htm. Here is a summary of where they are currently found:

Diphtheria. This disease is more prominent outside the United States. If you plan to travel and mingle with the natives for extended periods, diphtheria protection is fairly important. Areas where diphtheria still occurs on a regular basis, according to the CDC Web site, are:

- Africa—Algeria, Egypt, and the sub-Saharan countries
- Central and South America—Brazil, Colombia, Dominican Republic, Ecuador, Haiti, and Paraguay
- Asia/South Pacific—Afghanistan, Bangladesh, Bhutan, Cambodia, China, India, Indonesia, Laos, Mongolia, Burma, Nepal, Pakistan, Papua New Guinea, Philippines, Thailand, and Vietnam
- Middle East—Iran, Iraq, Syria, Turkey, and Yemen
- Europe—Albania and all countries of the former Soviet Union

Tetanus. If your child is injured in a Third World country, away from good medical care (and a sterile tetanus shot!), and is already vaccinated for tetanus, it is reassuring to know you don't have to worry. But if your child is not vaccinated for tetanus, realize that international travel in and of itself doesn't increase your child's risk of catching tetanus; it's not as if the soil in South America has more tetanus living in it than U.S. soil. (Or does it? That would be an interesting science fair project.)

Pertussis. Pertussis may be more common in Third World countries, but it is also fairly common in the United States, so traveling doesn't increase your child's risk of catching pertussis by much. However, if an infant or young child becomes seriously ill with pertussis while in a Third World country, the lack of good medical care may pose a risk.

Options to consider when getting this vaccine

Compare the aluminum content of the various brands. If possible, use one with a lower amount of aluminum. If you wish to limit your baby's aluminum exposure, you can choose to get only one aluminum-containing vaccine at a time.

Also, as mentioned on page 32, two brands use cow tissue extract and one doesn't. If exposure to animal tissues worries you (see pages 191 to 193 for more information), you may want to choose the brand that doesn't use cow extract. That same brand also contains a smaller dose of pertussis components.

You can choose to get the DTaP vaccine in combination with two other vaccines. Pediarix (GlaxoSmithKline) is a combination of the DTaP (Infanrix brand, page 33), the hep B (Engerix-B brand, page 54), and the polio vaccines. This one shot saves your baby from two other simultaneous injections, and the overall ingredients and manufacturing steps are similar to the separate vaccines made by GlaxoSmithKline. (See page 75 for an explanation of Pediarix's polio component.)

Another combination vaccine is Pentacel (Sanofi Pasteur). This vaccine has been in use in Canada for many years and has just been approved for use in the United States. It combines HIB with DTaP and polio all in one injection. Whereas most combo vaccines are just a sum of their individual parts, it is unclear whether or not this is the case with Pentacel because the product insert doesn't give details on how the vaccine is manufactured. It does state that the HIB component is the ActHIB brand. But the polio and DTaP components come from a combined vaccine called Quadracel, which isn't available in the United States. The Quadracel product insert doesn't list details on how the vaccine is made. It simply lists what all the final ingredients are. It doesn't state whether the DTaP components are made like Sanofi Pasteur's Daptacel brand or their Tripedia brand. The polio component is listed as a diploid cell origin polio vaccine, which is different from the Ipol brand of polio vaccine made by Sanofi Pasteur that we commonly use in the United States. The bottom line on Pentacel is that I can't determine exactly how it is made. But the product insert does list the final ingredients:

- HIB sugars bound to tetanus toxoid (see ActHIB, page 6, to see how this component is made)
- Proteins and toxins from the broken-up pertussis germs, and diphtheria and tetanus toxoids
- Polio virus (inactivated whole germs)
- Aluminum phosphate—1500 micrograms (which is only 330 micrograms of actual aluminum)
- 2-phenoxyethanol
- Polysorbate 80
- Cow serum (the liquid part of a cow's blood)
- Formaldehyde in trace amounts
- Traces of 2 antibiotics

My best guess is that this combo vaccine most closely resembles a mix of Sanofi Pasteur's ActHIB, Tripedia, and polio vaccines.

A third option to decrease the number of injections is the Tri-HIBit vaccine (Sanofi Pasteur), a combination of DTaP and HIB

(Tripedia and ActHIB brands) for the eighteen-month dose only (see page 12 for more details).

For more on combo vaccines, see page 153.

SEPARATE TETANUS AND DIPHTHERIA/TETANUS VACCINES

Some people prefer to get a separate tetanus (T) vaccine or the diphtheria/tetanus vaccine (DT or dT) instead of the DTaP. There are various reasons for this. Some parents choose not to give their infants the DTaP vaccine but decide to give their kids T or DT when they are older for tetanus protection. Another reason is that kids who react to the DTaP vaccine are thought to be most sensitive to the P component, and parents may decide to continue with the DT or plain T vaccine for tetanus coverage. Three doses of this vaccine are needed to get full protection. The second dose is given two months after the first, and the third dose is six to twelve months after the first.

Tetanus vaccine (Sanofi Pasteur)

The T vaccine is designed for those people who want only T protection against tetanus (such as an injured person who needs a tetanus shot). It is approved for use in kids age seven and older and for adults. (Doctors can administer it at any age; it just isn't officially approved for younger kids yet.) The manufacturing is similar to the tetanus component of the Tripedia brand of the DTaP vaccine, except that cow heart muscle extract is used to nourish the tetanus germs instead of the regular cow tissue extract used in the DTaP. The final ingredients are:

- Tetanus toxoid
- Aluminum—250 micrograms

- Saline solution
- Formaldehyde—less than 0.02 percent
- Mercury—less than 0.3 micrograms. It is used during manufacturing, but it is then filtered out. A very tiny amount remains, but it's less than 1 percent of what used to be there. Be aware, however, that Sanofi Pasteur also makes this vaccine in a 15-dose vial with mercury (25 micrograms). This form is less expensive. Be sure your doctor or ER uses the low-mercury single-dose vials.

DT vaccine (Sanofi Pasteur)

The "big D, big T" vaccine is designed for infants and children up to age seven. It shouldn't be used for older kids because they may react to the high D component (the dT discussed below has less of the diphtheria vaccine and is used for older kids and adults). Manufacturing is similar to that of the D and T components of the DTaP (Tripedia brand). Ingredients include:

- Diphtheria and tetanus toxoids
- Aluminum—170 micrograms
- Saline solution
- Formaldehyde—less than 0.02 percent
- Mercury—less than 0.3 micrograms. Sanofi Pasteur used to make this vaccine in a 10-dose vial with mercury (25 micrograms). This form was less expensive. Be sure your doctor or ER uses the low-mercury single-dose vials instead of any DT left over from a 10-dose vial.

dT vaccine (called "Decavac"–Sanofi Pasteur)

The "little d, big T" vaccine is designed for older children and adults (ages seven and up). There is less of the diphtheria component in this shot than in the DT or DTaP vaccine. The components are similar to those used in the D and T components of the DTaP (Tripedia brand). Ingredients include:

- Diphtheria and tetanus toxoids
- Aluminum—280 micrograms
- Saline solution
- Formaldehyde—less than 0.02 percent
- Mercury—less than 0.3 micrograms

Another company (Massachusetts Biologic Labs, distributed by General Injectables and Vaccines) makes a form of adult dT vaccine in large 15-dose vials with mercury. This company manufactures vaccines mainly for the state of Massachusetts. I have been unable to obtain the product insert to examine the details on how much mercury, but I believe it may be the full mercury dose. The bottom line on the dT is, if it's a single-dose vial, you know you're getting only trace amounts of mercury.

THE WAY I SEE IT

There are three diseases involved with this vaccine. All are serious, but only one, pertussis, is common in the United States. With pertussis so prevalent, this vaccine is very important. Infant fatalities do occur. The one drawback is the ingredient list, although, thankfully, the actual amounts of these chemicals are like a drop in a bucket—and a very small drop in a big bucket. Vaccination rates for DTaP must remain high if we are to keep pertussis at bay.

I've never seen any diphtheria or tetanus in my office, but I sure do see my fair share of pertussis—at least one case each month. And virtually all of these are in unvaccinated kids. I've had to hospitalize a few young babies, but fortunately they pulled through without any trouble. I consider this an important vaccine for infants and toddlers.

What about the newly recommended teenage and adult booster doses of Tdap? This is a good idea from a public health standpoint. Many cases of infant pertussis are caused by exposure to infected adults. Vaccinating our entire population should dramatically decrease infant fatalities. However, vaccinating grown-ups isn't an easy task. Most of us are big chickens when it comes to needles. Add to that the fact that the disease isn't a serious one beyond childhood and it's going to be hard to convince teens and adults to keep up with this shot.

4

Hepatitis B Disease and the Hep B Vaccine

WHAT IS HEP B?

Given that there's a hepatitis B, you're probably wondering if there was an A before it. Wonder no longer. There is a hepatitis A, as well as a C, D, E, and G. (What happened to F? I don't know.) We have vaccines for hep A (chapter 9) and hep B only. Hep B is a sexually transmitted virus that causes liver damage and sometimes liver failure. It can be fatal. Besides being transmitted through unprotected sex, hep B can also be passed on by the sharing of IV drug needles, the use of improperly sterilized tattoo needles, or an accidental stick with an infected needle. So any baby who participates in one of the above-mentioned risky activities could catch hepatitis B.

Now, it doesn't make sense to vaccinate babies for an STD, so you're probably thinking there must be more to the story. There is. Hep B can be acquired from a blood transfusion. Donated blood units are carefully tested for all kinds of diseases, but very rarely hepatitis B sneaks through. This is thought to occur in about 1 in every 65,000 to 500,000 blood units.

The Hepatitis B Vaccine
American Academy of Pediatrics
2007 Recommended Vaccine Schedule

Birth	**Hep B**
1 month	**Hep B**
2 months	HIB, Pc, DTaP, Rotavirus, Polio
4 months	HIB, Pc, DTaP, Rotavirus, Polio
6 months	HIB, Pc, DTaP, Rotavirus, **Hep B,** Flu
1 year	MMR, Chickenpox, Hep A
15 months	HIB, Pc
18 months	DTaP, Polio, Hep A, Flu
2 years	Flu
3 years	Flu
4 years	Flu
5 years	DTaP, Polio, MMR, Flu, Chickenpox
12 years	Tdap, Meningococcal, HPV (3 doses, girls only)

Theoretically, hep B can be transmitted also by contact with the saliva of an infected individual, but this is virtually unheard of. Also, if the blood of an infected person got on someone else, it could move through a cut or scrape and infect the person. Anyone living with an infected family member for many years is potentially at risk, since sooner or later they are likely to have close contact with the person's blood. The hep B virus can survive outside a person (such as on a toothbrush or razor) for one week. It is killed by disinfectant cleaning solutions with at least 10 percent bleach.

Finally, hep B can be passed from an infected mother to her baby during the birth process as the baby is exposed to the mom's blood and body fluids (the placenta protects the baby during pregnancy).

So, even though babies aren't sexually active, there are a few ways babies and children can catch hep B. Fortunately these occurrences are extremely rare.

Hep B is diagnosed with a blood test. Symptoms include abdominal pain, jaundice (yellow eyes and skin), vomiting, diarrhea, and fatigue.

IS HEP B COMMON?

This is a very difficult question to answer. On the one hand, there are the number of actual reported cases, and on the other hand, there are the number of suspected cases that go unrecognized in our population. Currently there are about 7500 new cases reported each year in the United States. About 6000 of these are in adults and about 1300 are in teens and college kids. Around 70 cases are reported each year in kids age five through fourteen, 30 cases in kids age one to four, and 30 cases in babies in the first year of life. So, this is a fairly rare disease in infants and children.

However, the total number of suspected cases of hep B in the United States is much higher, somewhere around 200,000 new cases each year.

Why is the number of reported cases so low compared with the number of suspected cases? And how can parents consider the risk of a disease with such a large discrepancy? To better understand this issue, let's take a look at hep B before vaccination began.

Twenty years ago a group of doctors from the Centers for Disease Control, several U.S. medical centers, and two pharmaceutical companies that make the hep B vaccine (GlaxoSmithKline and Merck) undertook the task of determining just how common the hep B infection was in infants and children. If they found that hep B was very common in kids, it would make sense to begin vaccination of all newborns. If the real incidence of hep B in kids was very low, however, there would be no reason to vaccinate all infants. Instead, we'd vaccinate just those born to a hep B–positive mom, and all teens and young adults (the highest-risk group).

The consensus of the researchers was that about 30,000 infants and children were being infected with this virus each year in the United States in the 1980s. However, the actual number of reported cases in all kids nine years and younger back then was only about 360 each year. Why were the estimates almost one hundred times higher than the reported cases? That is the $100,000 question.

Here is how the researchers came up with their estimate. (This is a very simplified explanation. For a detailed look at their research, you can examine the actual studies. See "Resources," page 264.) They did several studies to try to estimate how common hep B was in children. First they started with the total number of suspected carriers of hep B in the United States. It was thought that there were about 1.25 million chronic carriers nationwide at any given time. Statistical analysis showed that in order to have that many chronic carriers, there must be about 200,000 new cases each year. Research indicated that many adult cases couldn't be traced back to a known source (such as a sexual partner, an infected mother at the time of birth, or high-risk behaviors). It was hypothesized that many of the adults might have contracted the disease as children, and experts feared that hep B might not be only a sexually transmitted disease. They worried that it was being passed easily to children through casual day-to-day contact (since then, this has been documented only a handful of times). They concluded that as many as 30,000 infants and children must be contracting hep B each year in order to add up to the estimated 200,000 new cases each year and the 1.25 million chronic cases living in the United States. It was then decided in 1991 that all babies should be vaccinated in order to decrease hep B in our population. These researchers were part of a very well-respected group—the leaders in their field. Very few doctors questioned their data (see "Resources," page 264, for an article by one who did).

What was the actual number of diagnosed and reported cases of hep B back then, before vaccination began? In adults there were only about 20,000 new cases each year (about one-tenth of the estimates). And as I mentioned, only about 360 infants and children nine years and younger were being diagnosed each year. So how did the researchers make the jump in their estimates and come up with 30,000 kids? One assumption they made was that since only about 10 percent of kids who catch hep B show symptoms right away and some suffer only minor flu symptoms that never get diagnosed as hepatitis and pass with very little trouble, these cases might be rarely found and reported until the child becomes very ill, which might not occur until they are young adults. If this is true, it could account for about 3600 infections each year in kids. But that is still far short of the estimated 30,000.

The fact that there were only 360 reported cases each year in kids before vaccination started probably comes as a surprise to most doctors. That's because we are trained to believe that there were about 30,000 cases each year. How do I know there were so few reported cases? This number was extremely hard to find. Virtually no reports I searched through from the past twenty years provide this number. Instead, they state the number of reported hep B infections as a rate per 100,000 population. I could never find an actual, straightforward number. Then I hit upon a *Morbidity and Mortality Weekly Report* (see "Resources," page 265) that states very clearly in a graph at the end of the paper that in the late 1980s and early 1990s, there was about 1 case for every 100,000 kids each year in our population of kids from birth through nine years. This was the only paper I could find that detailed this number in the kids' population only. According to the U.S. Census Bureau, there were about 36 million kids in that age group in 1990. This comes out to about 360 cases reported in kids from birth through age nine each year. In the preceding paragraph, I conceded that you could multiply this number by ten (since only about 10 percent of childhood cases show symptoms) and come up with an approximate 3600 cases each year of kids who are hep B positive. But I still can't find a logical way to increase this number to 30,000. And remember, now that infant vaccination has been in place for over fifteen years, we have only about 130 confirmed cases of hep B each year in kids from birth to fourteen years.

So, having said all that, we come back to the question, is hep B common? In infants and children it is extremely rare. It occurs mainly in adults. Occasionally a baby may catch it from an infected mom at the time of birth, but treatment usually prevents this (see below). Some cases may occur in children who have no risk factors for hep B, but whether or not this really happens, and how often it may happen, is unknown. Ever since vaccination of infants and adults began, the number of all cases of hep B has decreased by about two-thirds.

IS HEP B SERIOUS?

Extremely. About 90 percent of babies who catch hep B during birth become chronically infected. They might not show symptoms for a while (many years or decades), but about 25 percent of them will develop liver cancer or liver failure eventually.

Kids who catch hep B during the toddler or preschool years have about a 35 percent chance of getting a chronic infection, and older kids and adults have only a 6 to 10 percent chance of developing a chronic disease. Immediate, symptomatic disease is more common in older age groups (compared with the babies), but the chance of liver failure or cancer is lower. There are an estimated four thousand deaths each year in the United States from liver failure or liver cancer due to hep B. These are virtually all among adults.

In a nutshell, infant and child hep B is often without symptoms for many years, but it is very serious when problems eventually begin. Teen and adult hep B is more often troublesome right away, but the long-term outlook is less severe.

IS HEP B TREATABLE?

No. There is no routine treatment available during the acute phase of the disease (when symptoms first begin). Fortunately in most adults it passes without much consequence. Unfortunately for kids, as discussed, it is more likely to cause long-term problems. If a child or adult continues to carry hep B as a chronic disease, treatment is available in the form of a medication similar to chemotherapy. About one-third of people are cured by this treatment, even kids.

Babies who are born to a mother who has hep B can be given a hep B antibody injection called HBIG to kill any viruses that pass into the baby during the birth process. This is an injection made up of hepatitis B antibodies filtered out of donated blood units from volunteers who have high antibody levels. This blood product is sterilized and filtered through various techniques. The injection contains the antibodies in a saline solution with polysorbate 80. It can be given to anyone who is exposed to blood known to contain the hep B virus.

WHEN IS THE HEP B VACCINE GIVEN?

It is given in three doses during the first year of life. The exact times used to vary among doctors. Some would start the series right at birth, and others would wait two months. The CDC and AAP have recently recommended the more precise schedule (see box), starting at birth. However, the only babies who actually need this birth dose are those born to a mom with hep B. Most babies can safely wait until they are two months of age. Parents should be aware that some hospitals give the hep B vaccine to babies without discussing it with the parents first. If you want to delay this shot, you should make sure your wishes are known to the medical staff at the hospital.

The current hep B vaccines became available in the early 1980s and vaccination for all infants began in the early 1990s.

HOW IS THE HEP B VACCINE MADE?

This is a very unique vaccine in that it is artificially engineered using advanced genetic techniques. The actual hep B virus is not in the final vaccine solution. There is no way to catch hep B from this vaccine.

A portion of DNA from the hep B virus is integrated into the DNA of some yeast cells that live in a solution of soy, sugar, amino acids, and minerals. The yeast cells then use this DNA to generate a protein that makes up the outer capsule of the hep B virus. The yeast cells are broken up, and the hep B protein is filtered out and purified. Aluminum is then added to help the vaccine work better. It is put into a saline solution.

The two brands of hep B vaccine vary slightly. Recombivax HB uses formaldehyde to help purify the vaccine. Engerix-B does not.

WHAT INGREDIENTS ARE IN THE FINAL VACCINE SOLUTION?

The Recombivax HB brand (Merck) contains:

- Hep B surface antigen (that's what the protein is called)
- Aluminum—250 micrograms per dose
- Saline solution
- Yeast proteins
- Formaldehyde—a residual amount. Although the Recombivax product insert does not list it as being part of the vaccine solution, the product insert for Comvax (see page 11) lists the residual amount of formaldehyde as 0.0004 percent of their final product, and since Comvax has Recombivax in it, I suspect the residual formaldehyde is there, just as it is in all other vaccines that use formaldehyde during manufacturing.

The Engerix-B brand (GlaxoSmithKline) contains:

- Hep B surface antigen
- Aluminum—250 micrograms per dose
- Saline solution
- Yeast proteins

Note: Both brands of the hep B vaccine used to contain mercury. When the government mandated around 1999 that mercury be filtered out of vaccines, the Recombivax brand stopped using mercury altogether. The Engerix-B brand began filtering out the mercury in 2002, but a tiny trace amount was left over (about 1 percent of what used to be there). In 2006 the Engerix-B brand stopped using mercury completely, and the current formulation is now 100 percent mercury free.

Are any of these ingredients controversial?

- Aluminum. See pages 193 to 206 for a discussion of aluminum.
- Formaldehyde. Although formaldehyde is toxic, the trace amount used is probably insignificant. See page 207 for more on the chemicals used in vaccines.

WHAT ARE THE SIDE EFFECTS OF THE HEP B VACCINE?

The standard side effects (see page 180) occur more frequently with the hep B vaccine than with many of the other shots. About 10 to 15 percent of people experience flu-like symptoms (fever, fatigue, weakness, irritability, headache, dizziness, diarrhea, and poor appetite).

Other reactions that have been reported include:

- Severe, life-threatening allergic reactions
- Severe rash
- Heart palpitations
- Minor liver damage
- Bleeding disorders (easy bruising, bleeding gums, blood in urine)
- Visual problems
- Hair loss
- Arthritis
- Lupus (the exact number of cases is unknown)

Neurological reactions, which are rare, include:

- Migraines
- Numbness, weakness, and nerve dysfunction
- Guillain-Barré syndrome
- Seizures
- Multiple sclerosis (has been reported to occur after the hep B vaccine; people with MS are cautioned in the Engerix package insert to get the vaccine only if their risk of exposure to hep B warrants it)

DO VACCINES REALLY *CAUSE* SIDE EFFECTS?

Each vaccine has a list of reported side effects. But it's important to realize that we don't know whether these reactions are caused by a vaccine or just happen to occur randomly within a month of a vaccine. Reactions don't have to be *proven* to have been caused by a vaccine before they are added to the list of side effects. There's an old saying in science: Temporality doesn't imply causality. Just because an event occurs after something doesn't mean that particular something caused that event. For example, when applied to vaccines, just because a child has a seizure one week after getting a particular vaccine doesn't prove that the seizure was related to the vaccine. However, if such a thing happens to numerous children, seizures still must be added to the list of *possible* side effects. So, as you read through my lists of side effects, keep in mind that there is no actual proof that most of these reactions are caused by vaccines.

On the other hand, this lack of proof has been heartbreaking for the many parents who feel their child did suffer a damaging reaction to a vaccine. Parents who have watched helplessly as their

SHOULD YOU GIVE YOUR BABY THE HEP B VACCINE?

Reasons to get this vaccine

I got this vaccine during medical school since I was going to come into contact with patients' blood. It is very important for any health care or emergency workers to get vaccinated with the hep B vaccine.

child developed neurologic problems within weeks of being vaccinated will probably always be 100 percent convinced that the vaccine caused the problems. The fact that neurologic reactions are listed in the product inserts lends credibility to their case.

There's an interesting story that I heard at a medical conference. A doctor was discussing a particular vaccine with some parents who were very concerned about the possible side effects. During the fifteen minutes that this discussion took place, their baby had a seizure. Now, if the parents had not delayed the shot by asking questions, their baby would have already gotten the shot when the seizure occurred. These parents would forever be absolutely convinced that the vaccine caused the seizure.

The truth is, sometimes infants and children develop medical problems for unknown reasons. Because of the frequency of infant vaccinations, most such problems occur within days or weeks of a vaccination. Although it can be highly suspected that the vaccine was the cause, it can't be proven. I'm sure the truth of the matter is somewhere in between causality and coincidence. Hopefully, someday we will have a better way to know for sure which side effects are truly vaccine related.

Of course, newborns with hep B–positive moms benefit greatly from the hep B antibody injection (HBIG) as well as from the vaccine to prevent transmission of the virus. All family members living with a hep B–positive person benefit from the vaccine.

The main controversy with the hep B vaccine is its universal use in infants. It does make sense that if all babies are vaccinated, a whole generation will grow up with protection from this STD and the disease should decrease in our general population. Furthermore, it appears that occasionally an infant or child may contract hep B from an unknown source (presumably contact with an infected person's saliva or blood), and vaccination prevents this from happening. One child in our practice stepped on a needle at a playground. He hadn't been vaccinated for hep B, and you can bet those parents were very scared. Thankfully, the needle tested negative for any infectious diseases.

Most parents feel that this vaccine is relatively safe because the manufacturing process and ingredients don't include any animal tissues.

Reasons some people choose not to get this vaccine

Some parents feel their babies and children aren't at risk of catching hep B. As you read on page 46, it is highly unlikely for hep B to be transmitted by casual day-to-day contact. Its main route of transmission is sexual.

Some of the reported side effects concern some parents.

Some parents decide to delay this shot in the early months while some of the more important shots (such as the pertussis and meningitis shots) are being done first.

Of course, when your teenage daughter comes home with her first boyfriend, riding on the back of a motorcycle, and she's impressed by the new tattoo on his arm and is thinking of getting one herself, it may be time to consider getting her this vaccine if she skipped it as a child.

Travel considerations

Vacation travel, as well as extended travel to visit family, conduct business, or work among native populations, does not put you at significant risk of catching this disease (as long as you don't get a tattoo or have intimate relations with anyone unknown to you). So this isn't a vaccine that anyone absolutely needs to get prior to travel. If you plan to live for six months or longer in a country with a high rate of hep B (keep reading) and are going to have considerable contact with the native population, vaccination should be considered.

You should be aware that certain populations around the world have a much higher incidence of hep B than we do in the United States. About 1 percent of the U.S. population carries hep B. Canada, western Europe, Australia, and the southern part of South America also have this low rate. However, the following areas have a much higher rate of hep B (about 12 percent of their population): Alaska (Native populations), Pacific Islands, China, Southeast Asia, eastern Europe, Central Asia, most of the Middle East, Africa, and the northern part of South America. Most cases in these areas are transmitted at the time of birth to infants. Countries not listed here have about 5 percent carriage rate.

Options to consider when getting this vaccine

Cautious parents may choose to separate this aluminum-containing vaccine from other shots that contain aluminum.

One option is to get the combo vaccine Comvax (Merck). It combines the HIB (PedVaxHIB brand) and hep B (Recombivax brand) vaccines in one shot. See page 11 for details. You can also choose Pediarix (GlaxoSmithKline), a combination of the DTaP, hep B, and polio vaccines. See page 40 for details. See page 153 for further discussion of combination shots. Children who delay the hep B vaccine until adolescence need only 2 doses if they use the Recombivax brand and get the shots between the ages of eleven and fifteen.

THE WAY I SEE IT

Even I have to admit that when it comes to the question, What diseases is a baby at risk of catching? hep B is very low on the list (unless you have one *very* rebellious baby). Yet, getting a whole generation of kids to grow up with hep B protection is a good way to minimize this disease in the future teen and adult population. So, do you get the shot early, while your child is young and can't voice an opinion? Or do you wait until she's older and getting closer to really needing the vaccine? (Not *your* kid, of course, I'm just talking in general terms.) It's not always easy to drag a teenager to the doctor to get one shot, let alone a series of three. Overall, this is an important vaccine from a public health standpoint, but it's not as critical from an individual point of view as most of the other infant vaccines.

5

Rotavirus Disease and the Rotavirus Vaccine

WHAT IS ROTAVIRUS?

Rotavirus is an intestinal virus that causes vomiting and diarrhea. An infant typically stays contagious for two to three weeks after symptoms begin. It is transmitted by contact with the stools or saliva of an infected person (another good reason to wash your hands after using the bathroom!). Unfortunately, rotavirus is resistant to common disinfectants and antibacterial hand soaps. It takes a strong antiseptic or alcohol solution to kill the germ. This makes it easily spread in day-care settings, where an adult changes numerous diapers, and kids share toys and food. Child-care providers should rinse their hands with an alcohol disinfectant solution between diaper changes, and disinfect toys appropriately every day.

Rotavirus is indistinguishable from the common stomach flu in the initial stages of the illness (fever, vomiting, and diarrhea). A clue that a baby may have rotavirus is that the diarrhea lasts more than just a few days (it can last for a few weeks in some cases) and is more frequent, watery, and foul smelling than

The Rotavirus Vaccine
American Academy of Pediatrics
2007 Recommended Vaccine Schedule

Birth	Hep B
1 month	Hep B
2 months	HIB, Pc, DTaP, **Rotavirus,** Polio
4 months	HIB, Pc, DTaP, **Rotavirus,** Polio
6 months	HIB, Pc, DTaP, **Rotavirus,** Hep B, Flu
1 year	MMR, Chickenpox, Hep A
15 months	HIB, Pc
18 months	DTaP, Polio, Hep A, Flu
2 years	Flu
3 years	Flu
4 years	Flu
5 years	DTaP, Polio, MMR, Flu, Chickenpox
12 years	Tdap, Meningococcal, HPV (3 doses, girls only)

diarrhea caused by stomach flu. (A baby may have as many as twelve diarrhea stools each day.) A stool test is available to diagnose rotavirus, but most doctors don't bother with this because the illness doesn't require specific treatment. Rotavirus can be caught more than once, but subsequent infections are usually milder.

IS ROTAVIRUS COMMON?

Yes. About 2 million people (mostly infants and children) are hospitalized each year worldwide for this disease. In the United States alone, about half a million doctor visits are made each year for rotavirus. It peaks here during late fall and winter. Interestingly, it usually starts in the southwestern states in November, spreads outward in an ever-widening circle, and eventually hits the East Coast by March. It then dwindles away as springtime blossoms. It is the most common cause of severe diarrhea in kids under age two, and by age three, most kids will have caught rotavirus at least once.

IS ROTAVIRUS SERIOUS?

Because it causes such persistent diarrhea and vomiting, severe dehydration is not uncommon. Each year in the United States, about fifty thousand kids are hospitalized for rotavirus. Between twenty and seventy infants and young children die each year nationwide because of dehydration from rotavirus. This is about one infant for every one thousand who are hospitalized. Worldwide, about half a million kids die each year because of this illness. Rotavirus is most severe in the first year of life. Cases beyond age two are less likely to cause trouble.

IS ROTAVIRUS TREATABLE?

No. There is no medication to combat rotavirus. Infants who are not significantly dehydrated usually do fine at home with the proper hydration measures. Taking a probiotic powder (such as acidophilus, available at a health food or vitamin store) can shorten the course of the disease. Avoiding cow's milk or cow's-milk formula for a few weeks can also help the diarrhea subside more quickly. Soy formula or soy milk can be used as an alternative during this time. Breast milk is the best hydration a baby can get.

Those who are significantly dehydrated can receive IV fluids in an ER and then be sent home. Infants who are severely dehydrated often need to stay in the hospital for a few days until the vomiting and diarrhea subside.

WHEN IS THE ROTAVIRUS VACCINE GIVEN?

The rotavirus vaccine is given as a liquid by mouth. There are two brands of the rotavirus vaccine, and they have different schedules.

The RotaTeq brand is given in a 3-dose series at two months, four months, and six months. The first dose should be given between six and twelve weeks of age, and the last dose should be completed by thirty-two weeks of age. The manufacturers studied the vaccine only when given within these specific time frames. They don't know how well the vaccine works or what the possible side effects are if the series is started later than twelve weeks of age or completed beyond thirty-two weeks of age. Until further research is done, this dosing schedule should be adhered to.

The Rotarix brand, which is likely to be available for use in late 2007, is a 2-dose series, the first given around two months, and the second around four months. At least one month should separate the two doses.

The rotavirus vaccine is currently the only oral vaccine in the vaccine schedule. If an infant spits out the RotaTeq brand, the company recommends it not be repeated (enough is usually swallowed for it to work). The makers of Rotarix say a replacement dose can be given if most of the first dose is spit out.

HOW IS THE ROTAVIRUS VACCINE MADE?

The process varies by manufacturer.

RotaTeq. Five different strains of rotavirus that were originally taken from infected humans and infected cows are used. The viruses are "cross-bred" genetically to increase their effectiveness for the vaccine. The viruses are then grown in a mix of monkey kidney cells (called VERO cells) nourished by fetal cow serum (blood from a cow fetus). Batches of the virus are filtered out from these cells and placed in a liquid solution (see the next section for ingredients).

Rotarix. This is a single strain of the most common human rotavirus strain. Since Rotarix has not yet been approved for use (as of late 2007), I am unable to find details on how it is made. I do know that the virus is grown in a culture of monkey kidney cells (similar to RotaTeq), and I do know what the final ingredients are (see the next section). I will post the details about the actual manufacturing process at www.TheVaccineBook.com when the product insert becomes available.

The viruses are whole and live when administered to patients. In fact, they are intended to multiply in the intestines of infants in order to create a mild infection that the body's immune system responds to so it can fight off the real infection if it ever hits.

The live viruses can come out in the diaper for up to fifteen days after the first dose. With RotaTeq, this occurs in 10 percent of babies but doesn't happen after the second or third dose. With Rotarix, preliminary reports indicate this may happen in up to 50 percent of babies and can continue for a few weeks after the second dose. It isn't known exactly how contagious postvaccination feces are, but some cases of virus transmission to a nonvaccinated baby have occurred. It's worth being especially careful about diaper-changing hygiene during this time.

WHAT INGREDIENTS ARE IN THE FINAL VACCINE SOLUTION?

The RotaTeq brand (Merck) contains:

- Five virus strains, live and whole
- Sucrose (a sugar)
- Sodium citrate, phosphate, and hydroxide (electrolyte chemicals)
- Polysorbate 80
- Cell culture media (the gel or liquid that the viruses sit in as they grow; specific ingredients aren't detailed)
- Traces of fetal cow blood

The Rotarix brand (GlaxoSmithKline) contains:

- Single virus strain, live and whole
- Sucrose (a sugar)
- Dextran
- Sorbitol (a sugar)
- Amino acids
- Dulbecco's Modified Eagle Medium (the solution that the virus is kept in for growth; details on it aren't listed in the PI)
- Calcium carbonate
- Xanthum gum
- Sterile water

Are any of these ingredients controversial?

- Monkey kidney cells (see page 192)
- Fetal cow blood (page 192)
- Polysorbate 80 (page 209)
- The use of live, genetically altered organisms is a worry to some people, even outside the food industry.

WHAT ARE THE SIDE EFFECTS OF THE ROTAVIRUS VACCINE?

Standard side effects (see page 180) were studied for forty-two days after each dose, and these reactions occurred at the same rate in infants who got the vaccine as those who got a placebo (nonvaccine oral solution). These reactions occured in 5 to 10 percent of infants in both groups.

Since the vaccine germs are intended to cause a mild intestinal infection, I would expect babies to experience some mild symptoms of rotavirus. Interestingly the research didn't show this any more than in the placebo group.

Two other reactions have been observed:

Seizures. These can occur after any vaccine, usually from a high fever, not from the vaccine itself. About one in every thirteen hundred rotavirus vaccine test subjects had a seizure. Seizures did occur almost twice as often in the vaccine group as in the placebo group. While this seems like a fairly small risk, this seizure rate is much higher than with most vaccines.

Intussusception. This is an intestinal complication in which part of the intestine "telescopes" into itself, creating a very serious and life-threatening blockage. An older version of the rotavirus vaccine, called RotaShield, was taken off the market in 1999 due to this side effect, so researchers have been diligently watching for this problem now that a different version of the vaccine has been developed. The older vaccine used a mix of human and rhesus monkey strains of rotavirus. It is not clear which components of this vaccine caused the problem, but some believe that monkey strains cause more reactions and inflammation in the intestines of humans than other strains, thus increasing the risk of complications. The two new vaccines use human and cow strains instead of monkey strains.

In the safety trial for the new vaccine, RotaTeq, out of 36,000 infants, 13 had intussusception within one year. Of the 36,000 infants who were given a placebo, 15 had this complication. In 2006, during the first several months of the new vaccine's use in the general population, 28 cases of intussusception occurred in infants after they were vaccinated. Some occurred within a day or two, and some as long as two months later. None of these cases were fatal, although half required surgery. This was after 3.5 million doses were distributed around the country (it is not known how many were actually given). However, the expected number of yearly cases of intussusception before the rotavirus vaccine was ever used was between 18 and 43 cases per 100,000 kids. There are numerous causes of intussusception that have nothing to do with vaccination. So, while this problem is being reported again with the rotavirus vaccine, the number of cases seems to be what we would expect to occur anyway. So far, vaccine policymakers recommend that the use of this vaccine continue—they see no greater risk of intussusception.

Symptoms of intussusception include extreme fussiness, vomiting, bloody stools, and episodes of intense abdominal pain. Infants often draw the knees up to the abdomen for several minutes while in pain, then relax into lethargy for several minutes as the pain subsides. The pain continues in waves like this that can last as long as thirty minutes at a time. This is considered an emergency and should be evaluated in an ER right away if you suspect your infant is having this reaction.

SHOULD YOU GIVE YOUR BABY THE ROTAVIRUS VACCINE?

Reasons to get this vaccine

Besides the flu, this is the most common of all the vaccine-preventable diseases right now. Since most children catch this illness during their first few years of life, it's not a question of *will* your child catch it, it's a matter of *when* will he catch it and *how severe* will it be. Getting this vaccine will decrease your child's chance of catching the disease. This can be a very serious disease for infants during the first year of life. The vaccine decreases the severity of the illness when it does strike.

Infants in day care are at high risk of catching this illness. Formula-fed infants are likely to suffer a more severe case.

Vaccinating all infants would help decrease and maybe someday eliminate this disease from our population.

Reasons some people choose not to get this vaccine

Some parents may worry because the older vaccine, RotaShield, had a small risk of intussusception. One of the new brands has been out for about a year now, and so far this risk doesn't seem to be an issue. The second brand is just about to hit the market, so we don't yet know about its risk. Some cautious parents may wait another year or two until this matter is studied further before they vaccinate their babies.

Infants who are breastfed and not in day care have a fairly low risk of catching this disease during the first year of life (when it is most risky), so some of their parents may choose to skip this vaccine.

As with all new vaccines, we don't yet know what all the side effects are. Some parents may want to wait until we do.

The animal products used to make this vaccine may also worry some parents. Although rotavirus is a very common disease, fatalities are rare in the United States.

Travel considerations

Rotavirus isn't more common in other countries. However, if a baby caught rotavirus while visiting a Third World country, the lack of quality health care would give the baby a higher risk of complications. Normal vacation travel probably isn't risky, but any unvaccinated baby visiting the native population in a developing country would be at risk. In tropical climates rotavirus is a year-round illness (as opposed to a winter disease here), so it can be caught anytime if your travels take you to lush green locations.

Options to consider when getting this vaccine

Since this is a live-virus vaccine, parents are urged to be cautious if their infant has a compromised immune system or is taking medications that suppress the immune system. This isn't listed as an absolute contraindication in the product insert, however.

Since this is a new vaccine, very cautious parents may decide to have their child get this vaccine by itself, without any other simultaneous shots.

THE WAY I SEE IT

This infection can be a real pain in the ... diaper area. It is extremely common. During my training years, I remember the hospital hallways would be overflowing with dehydrated babies and worried parents because of this bug. Fortunately, the actual number of fatalities is low in the United States. Perhaps twenty years from now we'll look back and say, "Remember the old days, when rotavirus was around?" Sure, the vaccine is new and the ingredients are a little odd, and this might give some parents pause. But this vaccine should help us get rid of rotavirus. I consider this a fairly important vaccine.

6

Polio Disease and the Polio Vaccine

WHAT IS POLIO?

Polio is a virus that is transmitted like the common cold or an intestinal flu. Most cases don't show any symptoms. Some people have a minor sore throat and fever. One in every 250 cases develops muscle weakness and paralysis. Polio can be caught only once in a lifetime.

IS POLIO COMMON?

Fortunately, no. There haven't been any cases of polio in the United States since 1985, when an immigrant came in with the disease. No U.S.-residing citizen has contracted wild polio (not caused by the vaccine) since 1979. The last case of wild polio in the entire Western Hemisphere was in 1991. There are a couple of thousand cases each year reported in several parts of Asia and Africa.

In 2005 an Amish person from Minnesota got an oral live-virus

The Polio Vaccine
American Academy of Pediatrics
2007 Recommended Vaccine Schedule

Birth	Hep B
1 month	Hep B
2 months	HIB, Pc, DTaP, Rotavirus, **Polio**
4 months	HIB, Pc, DTaP, Rotavirus, **Polio**
6 months	HIB, Pc, DTaP, Rotavirus, Hep B, Flu
1 year	MMR, Chickenpox, Hep A
15 months	HIB, Pc
18 months	DTaP, **Polio,** Hep A, Flu
2 years	Flu
3 years	Flu
4 years	Flu
5 years	DTaP, **Polio,** MMR, Flu, Chickenpox
12 years	Tdap, Meningococcal, HPV (3 doses, girls only)

polio vaccine overseas (we no longer use this live-virus vaccine in the United States). The live polio virus from the vaccine then spread from that person to a few unvaccinated children within that Amish community. Since these cases were caused by the vaccine and did not occur naturally, we still consider the United States polio free since 1985.

IS POLIO SERIOUS?

Yes, it can be. While most cases are harmless, some unfortunate individuals become paralyzed. It is usually temporary, but two-thirds of them suffer permanent muscle weakness. Most often it is not fatal.

IS POLIO TREATABLE?

No. The person is supported with breathing machines in an ICU for several weeks until the paralysis wears off. Today's older generation will never forget the rows upon rows of "iron lung" machines for polio victims.

WHEN IS THE POLIO VACCINE GIVEN?

We give the injected polio vaccine at two months, four months, eighteen months, and five years. The third dose, however, can be given at any time between six months and eighteen months, and the fourth dose can be given at any time between four and six years. The injected polio vaccine has been around for many decades.

HOW IS THE POLIO VACCINE MADE?

Ipol (Sanofi Pasteur) is the only brand used in the United States. First, a culture of monkey kidney cells is nourished with calf serum (the liquid portion of the cow's blood). The monkey kidney cells are then removed from the cow serum, and three strains of the polio virus (their origin is unknown, but presumably they came from individuals infected decades ago) are mixed with the monkey cells in a culture medium called M-199, which is a saline solution with vitamins, amino acids, sucrose, glutamate, and human albumin (proteins filtered out of donated human blood units). Three antibiotics are also mixed in to keep the solution sterile. The polio virus uses the monkey kidney cells to multiply. Batches of the virus are then removed from the kidney cells, thoroughly purified through several steps, then warmed for twelve days in a solution of formalin to inactivate the virus. Formaldehyde and 2-phenoxyethanol are added as preservatives.

This vaccine contains the whole virus, but it is inactivated, so there is no way for it to infect people.

You may have heard that the polio vaccine can actually cause paralysis. This was true of the old vaccine, which was given as a live-virus liquid by mouth. Thankfully, it was taken off the U.S. market in the early 2000s. This was because about eight children each year in the United States were being paralyzed by the vaccine. Now we use only the injected, inactivated form, so there are no longer any paralytic reactions to the vaccine.

WHAT INGREDIENTS ARE IN THE FINAL VACCINE SOLUTION?

The final product contains:

- Three inactivated virus strains
- M-199 culture medium (saline, vitamins, amino acids, sucrose, glutamate, and human albumin), added at the end of the process to dilute the virus. (Those of you who are reading the package inserts yourself will notice that the polio PI lists M-199 in the manufacturing process but doesn't elaborate on what the ingredients of M-199 are. In the MMR vaccine product insert, the ingredients of M-199 are given in detail. That is how I am able to list the details of M-199 here. (You really can stop trying to decipher the PIs on your own—I've done my homework on this.)
- 2-phenoxyethanol—about 0.5 percent of the vaccine solution
- Formaldehyde—about 0.02 percent of the vaccine solution
- Residual amounts of three antibiotics
- Traces of the calf serum, left over in the vaccine solution—1 part per million

Are any of these ingredients controversial?

- Baby cow blood serum
- Human albumin (blood proteins). This is also in the vaccine solution (a component of the M-199 culture medium).
- Glutamate. Part of the M-199 culture medium, glutamate is a component of MSG (monosodium glutamate). See page 209 for more information.
- Formaldehyde and 2-phenoxyethanol. These two chemicals do have some toxicity when used in high amounts. The trace amount used here is probably harmless, but see pages 209 and 210 for a more extensive discussion.
- Monkey kidney cells. This is the most controversial aspect of this vaccine. See page 191 for a discussion of the safety of using human and animal tissues and blood products to make vaccines.

WHAT ARE THE SIDE EFFECTS OF THE POLIO VACCINE?

The standard side effects (see page 180) don't occur as often with the polio vaccine as with other vaccines.

The only unusual reaction that has been reported is Guillain-Barré syndrome. It has been reported after various vaccines, so the polio vaccine is not unique in this. This reaction is extremely rare with the polio vaccine (the exact number of cases is unknown). See page 181 for more on GBS.

SHOULD YOU GIVE YOUR BABY THE POLIO VACCINE?

Reasons to get this vaccine

Universal vaccination against polio has eliminated this disease from North America, Europe, South America, and Australia (and I guess Antarctica as well, so you're safe to go there). Until polio is eradicated from the world (like smallpox was nearly forty years ago), there is always the potential that polio could take hold within our country again if people don't get this vaccine.

The side effect profile is one of the safest of all vaccines.

Some people worry about immigrants bringing in polio (although this hasn't happened in twenty-five years), so they feel better if their child gets vaccinated.

Reasons some people choose not to get this vaccine

The use of monkey kidney cells, cow serum, and human blood proteins gives some parents pause. Since polio doesn't exist in our country, some parents feel safe about skipping this vaccine. The chance that an unvaccinated child will catch polio while living in the United States is very close to zero. Some parents do wish to protect their children from polio along with the rest of our population, but they worry about adding this vaccine in with all the other shots during the early infant years. These parents often vaccinate their kids as they get older.

Travel considerations

Obviously, if you are not vaccinated, it would be risky to go live or take an extended vacation in those countries in Africa and Asia where polio still occurs. The four main countries in which polio is still considered endemic (constantly present in a specific population or area) are India, Pakistan, Afghanistan, and Nigeria (Niger and Egypt were taken off the endemic list in 2006, but some cases continue to strike there). In 2003–2004 an epidemic of polio spread through the entire sub-Saharan region of Africa. People who were not immunized as babies should get at least two shots of the polio vaccine before traveling to these countries.

Areas of the world where polio is considered eradicated include the Western Hemisphere, the Western Pacific region (including China), and Europe. Please note that the list of countries that continue to struggle with polio changes every few years. You can find current information on polio on the CDC Web site, www.cdc.gov/travel/diseases.htm.

Options to consider when getting this vaccine

There is a combination vaccine called Pediarix (GlaxoSmith-Kline), a mix of the DTaP, hep B, and polio vaccines. See page 40 for a detailed discussion of this vaccine. Choosing this one shot saves your baby from two other simultaneous injections. Interestingly, the manufacturing process for the polio component in this triple shot is very similar to that in Sanofi Pasteur's plain polio vaccine, described in this chapter, except that Glaxo-

SmithKline doesn't use human blood proteins (albumin). However, Glaxo doesn't offer its polio as an individual vaccine.

Another combination vaccine is Pentacel (Sanofi Pasteur), a mix of the polio, DTaP, and HIB vaccines, which has been used in Canada for many years and has just been approved for use in the United States. See page 40 for details on this vaccine.

For further discussion of all combo vaccines, see page 153.

THE WAY I SEE IT

Since polio was eradicated from the United States more than twenty years ago and isn't even found on this half of the planet, it is safe to say that we don't give this vaccine in order to protect each individual child from catching polio. Rather, we do it to protect our nation as a whole in the event an outbreak does occur (cue background patriotic music, like "America the Beautiful"). Although the ingredients may seem a little odd, we don't see many side effects from this shot. If we stop using this vaccine, polio may come back. Anyone who is over fifty knows just how scary that would be (". . . purple mountains' majesty, da da da dum di day . . ."—I can't remember the words). For younger people, polio might not seem like a reality. When parents tell me they want to skip the polio shot for their child, I tell them, "Okay. Your child is almost guaranteed not to catch polio. You better just pray that not too many of your neighbors make the same choice, or in ten years we may all be in trouble." While I realize some parents think it isn't critical for infants to receive the polio vaccine during the early years (compared with the vaccines for diseases like pertussis and meningitis), I consider this vaccine very important from a public health viewpoint. Until the whole world is polio free, ongoing vaccination will help keep our nation protected "from sea to shining sea."

7

Measles, Mumps, and Rubella Diseases and the MMR Vaccine

Measles

WHAT IS MEASLES?

Measles is a virus that travels throughout the body and causes a fever, rash (red, round bumps and spots all over the body), runny nose, and cough. The rash can look similar to rashes symptomatic of other diseases, so it's not easy for a doctor, much less a parent, to recognize. A blood test can be done to confirm the diagnosis. Measles is transmitted like the common cold, and infection usually creates lifelong immunity.

IS MEASLES COMMON?

Not anymore. In the early part of the twentieth century, there were about a million cases every year in the United States. Now we have only 50 to 100 cases reported each year. The number of actual cases is probably higher than this, since not all cases are

The MMR Vaccine
American Academy of Pediatrics
2007 Recommended Vaccine Schedule

Birth	Hep B
1 month	Hep B
2 months	HIB, Pc, DTaP, Rotavirus, Polio
4 months	HIB, Pc, DTaP, Rotavirus, Polio
6 months	HIB, Pc, DTaP, Rotavirus, Hep B, Flu
1 year	**MMR,** Chickenpox, Hep A
15 months	HIB, Pc
18 months	DTaP, Polio, Hep A, Flu
2 years	Flu
3 years	Flu
4 years	Flu
5 years	DTaP, Polio, **MMR,** Flu, Chickenpox
12 years	Tdap, Meningococcal, HPV (3 doses, girls only)

diagnosed or reported. Officially measles is no longer considered endemic in the United States (constantly present in a specific population or area at considerable levels). Measles now occurs only as isolated outbreaks, such as the one that occurred in May 2005 with 33 cases in one geographic area.

IS MEASLES SERIOUS?

Usually not. Most cases, especially in children, pass in a week or so without any trouble. However, approximately 1 in 1000 cases is fatal. Back when measles was common, there were a number of deaths each year in the United States. Now that measles is rare, many years go by without any fatalities.

Measles (as well as mumps and rubella) can infect various internal organs and cause a number of complications. These are all extremely rare. The possible complications from measles, mumps, or rubella are very similar to the side effects of the vaccines themselves. (See pages 180 to 183 for a list of these possible problems.) Rarely, measles can infect the brain and cause brain damage.

IS MEASLES TREATABLE?

No. The illness must run its course. If a child becomes seriously ill and is hospitalized, high-dose vitamin A therapy can be used to lessen the duration and severity of the disease.

Mumps

WHAT IS MUMPS?

Mumps is a virus similar to measles. It causes fever, rash, and swelling of the saliva glands in the cheeks (right in front of the ears). Rarely, the virus infects internal organs. The swelling of the cheeks is usually the most telling sign of mumps, and a blood test can be done to confirm the diagnosis. It is transmitted like the common cold, and once you catch mumps, you are protected for life.

IS MUMPS COMMON?

No. In the past decade only about 250 cases have been reported each year in the United States. Early in the twentieth century, there were several hundred thousand cases each year.

In the spring of 2006 a mumps outbreak occurred among Iowa college students and spread to several surrounding states. More than 3000 cases were eventually reported, the largest outbreak in over twenty years. About twenty victims were hospitalized, but none of the cases were fatal. Most of the infected people had been vaccinated during childhood, but immunity from the vaccine usually wears off by adulthood, so this wasn't a case of vaccine failure. It occurred simply because adults don't get booster shots for mumps (we're all too chicken!). This mini epidemic should run its course, and things will settle back down to normal.

IS MUMPS SERIOUS?

No. In fact, most kids who have mumps have some fever and a slight rash but not enough for anyone to worry about or even make a diagnosis (thus, the true number of cases is probably higher than 250 each year, since many cases go unrecognized). For teens and adults, however, mumps can be more serious. Males may have sore, swollen testicles, and men or women can have arthritis, kidney problems, heart problems, or nervous system dysfunction. Very rarely, the disease can make adults (men and women) sterile.

IS MUMPS TREATABLE?

No. Like measles, it must run its course.

Rubella

WHAT IS RUBELLA?

Like measles and mumps, rubella is a virus that causes a fever and rash (red, round bumps and spots all over the body). It can also cause aching joints and swelling of the glands behind the ears and in the neck. In children the disease is so mild that it often goes unnoticed. A blood test can confirm the diagnosis. It is transmitted like the common cold and a person catches rubella only once in a lifetime.

If rubella is so mild, why vaccinate for it? We do it because if a pregnant woman catches rubella (she would be susceptible if she'd never had the disease or if the rubella vaccine she got as a child had worn off), it can infect her fetus and cause birth defects. So, we vaccinate kids to protect pregnant teachers and mothers and their soon-to-be-born babies. If a pregnant woman is exposed to rubella, blood testing can be done to see if she actually caught the virus, but the full effects on the fetus, if any, can't be known until the baby is born. Rubella is most risky to a fetus during the first trimester and only somewhat risky in the second trimester. There is no risk during the third trimester.

IS RUBELLA COMMON?

No. There used to be about 100,000 cases per year, but with universal vaccination this decreased to about 250 cases each year in recent decades. In the past few years, only about 20 cases have been reported each year in the United States. Rubella is now so rare, it is considered effectively eliminated from the U.S. population, thanks to our nation's vaccine program. There may be more cases than are being reported, since it is such a mild disease and the younger generation of doctors may not even recognize it when they see it.

How many babies are born each year with rubella-induced birth defects (called congenital rubella syndrome, or CRS)? Over the past two decades about 10 babies have been born with CRS each year. In the past few years this has declined to only about 3 babies each year. In 1990 there was an unexplained jump in rubella to 1125 reported cases. This resulted in 34 babies born with rubella birth defects each year for the next two years. This illustrates what could happen if rubella came back as a common disease.

IS RUBELLA SERIOUS?

No. As stated above, it's virtually unrecognizable in children, and usually harmless for adults. It is not a fatal disease. However, some of the birth defects in a fetus are permanent (hearing loss, heart, eye, and brain defects, and growth problems). Rubella can also cause stillbirth.

IS RUBELLA TREATABLE?

No treatment is given to infected people. The virus just has to run its course. Even a pregnant woman doesn't get treated. Most of a baby's birth defects are untreatable, although some may be correctable with surgery.

WHEN IS THE MMR VACCINE GIVEN?

It is given at twelve months of age, with a booster dose at five years. This booster can be given anytime between four and six years. Why not give both shots earlier? The MMR vaccine is a live-virus vaccine. That means the viruses in the vaccine are whole and living. They need a more mature immune system to recognize them. A one-year-old will get better immunity from the vaccine than a younger infant would. In fact, if your baby gets the shot before his first birthday, some states don't count it as being valid. One advantage of a live-virus vaccine is that a person needs only one initial shot for it to work (with a follow-up booster years later), instead of an initial series of three or four shots. The booster is needed because the first shot wears off after several years in some people, and it helps ensure these people are protected. An alternative approach would be to do blood testing on everybody every few years, and give the booster only to those who have lost their immunity. But you can imagine how complicated that would be.

For parents who decide against the MMR vaccine for their baby but want their child to get it later, only one shot is needed if it's delayed until after age four. Some states, however, will require such children to get two shots.

Measles, mumps, and rubella vaccines have been in use for several decades, but the current triple MMR vaccine, called MMR II, has been in use since the early 1990s.

HOW IS IT MADE?

Hold on to your seats. This may be the most complicated manufacturing process so far.

I could not determine where the measles and mumps viruses originally came from, but they probably came from infected individuals many decades ago. The rubella virus was originally taken from an infected aborted fetus in the 1960s.

The measles and mumps viruses are nourished for years in a culture of chicken embryo cells. The rubella virus is nourished in a culture of human lung cells. Each of these tissue cultures is contained in a solution of saline, amino acids, vitamins, serum from a cow fetus (the liquid portion of the cow's blood), sugar, gelatin, neomycin (an antibiotic), and, finally, human albumin (a protein filtered out of donated human blood units).

The cell cultures, cow fetus serum, and human blood proteins are tested to make sure no errant infectious germs are present. Then the three viruses are removed from the cultures in batches and put into the vaccine solution. They are alive but weakened so they won't (usually) cause an actual infection when injected.

Why is the process so complicated? The numerous nutrients are needed to keep the chicken embryo cells and human lung cells alive so that the viruses can keep using the cells to multiply.

WHAT INGREDIENTS ARE IN THE FINAL VACCINE SOLUTION?

- The three viruses
- Saline solution, sugars, and gelatin
- Human albumin (blood proteins)
- Residual cow fetus serum (< 1 part per million)
- Neomycin (an antibiotic)
- Traces of chick embryo proteins
- "Other buffer and media ingredients" (details are not listed in the product insert)

Are any of these ingredients controversial?

Instead of the various chemicals used in some vaccines, MMR has some unusual human and animal tissue components:

- Human albumin
- Cow fetus serum
- Chick embryo proteins

See page 191 for a detailed discussion of the use of human and animal tissues in vaccines.

WHAT ARE THE SIDE EFFECTS OF THE MMR VACCINE?

Common reactions to the MMR vaccine are general aches, mild rash, and fever. These sometimes occur up to two weeks later and are not contagious. Because they are so common (about one in twenty children experiences them), be sure you don't have any big plans over the two weeks following this vaccination that might be interrupted if your child isn't feeling well.

Below is a list of some of the more troublesome side effects reported on the product insert. These effects can also happen with the natural diseases themselves. These complications are all rare:

- Measles infection (caused by the occasional inadequately weakened virus in the vaccine)
- Flu-like symptoms
- Inflammation of the blood vessels
- Inflamed pancreas
- Diabetes
- Bleeding disorders (low platelet levels) and bruising throughout the body (I have seen this reaction twice in my office over the ten years I've been a pediatrician.)
- Rubella infection
- Allergic reactions
- Joint and muscle soreness
- Life-threatening rash (Stevens-Johnson syndrome)
- Mumps infection, including mumps-like swelling of the saliva glands in the cheeks, inflamed testicles, and meningitis. The package insert states that research shows "a causal relationship between mumps vaccine and mumps meningitis" (see "Resources," page 261, for several articles from *The Lancet* that discuss this side effect).
- Rare deaths from unknown causes

Nervous system dysfunctions listed include the following:

- Eye inflammation and visual dysfunction
- Nerve inflammation and dysfunction
- Deafness (due to dysfunction of the hearing nerve)
- Seizures due to fever
- Seizures not associated with fever
- Guillain-Barré syndrome (muscle weakness and paralysis; see page 181)

Two particular reactions are highlighted in the product insert:

Chronic arthritis. The product insert cites three research studies (see "Resources," page 262) that have shown a 12 to 26 percent chance that teenage and adult women who get the MMR or the plain rubella vaccine may experience significant arthritis for days, months, or, rarely, years. Infants, children, and adult men don't seem to have this risk.

Encephalitis and encephalopathy. Encephalitis is inflammation (swelling and irritation) of the brain tissue. This is usually brief and harmless. When it is severe or prolonged (occurring for days), it can lead to dysfunction or damage of the brain tissue, known as encephalopathy. A related condition called subacute sclerosing panencephalitis, or SSPE (and you thought "intussusception" was a tough one to say!), occurs when this reaction is mild, yet chronic, and the brain gradually deteriorates over many years. See page 181 for more on these reactions.

The product insert states, "The data suggest the possibility that some of these cases [of encephalitis] may have been caused by measles vaccines," and, "After 200 million doses . . . serious events such as encephalitis and encephalopathy continue to be rarely reported." Another source (see "Resources," page 261) states that encephalitis occurs once every million doses. To my knowledge, no precise accounting of the statistical chance of this reaction has been determined for sure.

SHOULD YOU GIVE YOUR BABY THE MMR VACCINE?

Reasons to get this vaccine

Measles is a disease with some possibly serious effects, and its fatality rate is something to consider (about 1 in 1000 cases; compare this with chickenpox's fatality rate, for example, which is only about 1 in 65,000 cases).

Mumps, while almost never fatal, can be a troublesome disease for teenagers and adults, with some serious effects.

Rubella, while harmless to children and adults alike, can cause birth defects or stillbirth. Vaccinating children limits the exposure to pregnant women.

Continued vaccination of all children helps keep these three diseases at low levels in our population.

Reasons some people choose not to get this vaccine

Measles is now extremely rare and in most cases harmless. The chance that a child will catch measles *and* be one of the rare fatalities is extremely low.

Mumps and rubella are mild diseases in children, and both are rare. Some parents simply don't worry about vaccinating for diseases that are both mild and rare.

Perhaps the main reason some parents worry about this vaccine is that the potential side effects, although rare, can be considerable when they do occur. The human and cow blood products used in manufacturing may also concern some parents.

Since some of the side effects of this vaccine involve the immune system, some families with a very strong history of autoimmune disorders (such as rheumatoid arthritis, lupus, and multiple sclerosis) worry that their babies may be more prone to autoimmune reactions to this vaccine. This worry is theoretical and hasn't been extensively researched.

Some families delay this shot for several years, then consider getting it when their kids approach the teenage years (measles and mumps are more severe diseases for teens and adults, anyway).

Travel considerations

Measles, mumps, and rubella are rare in the United States, but this is not true internationally. Vacation travel isn't very risky, but if you are planning to mingle with the natives for several weeks, you might want to investigate whether these diseases are common where you are going.

Measles is still very common in Africa, East Asia, and most Third World countries. Even some developed countries in Europe and Asia still have a problem with measles. Mumps and rubella are both fairly common in most other countries of the world, even developed ones. Good data that list exactly which countries do and don't have a problem with mumps and rubella aren't readily available.

For up-to-date travel information on these diseases, visit the CDC Web site, www.cdc.gov/travel/diseases.htm.

Options to consider when getting this vaccine

Since this is a live-virus vaccine, it may be beneficial to make sure a baby's overall health and immune system are at their peak prior to the shot. Make sure your baby hasn't been on antibiotics in the past few weeks and isn't currently experiencing allergic or infectious diarrhea. Taking vitamin C and vitamin A before and after this shot is recommended by some doctors to help the body guard against some side effects (see page 190 for a more detailed discussion).

The chickenpox vaccine is routinely given at one year of age, at the same time as the MMR vaccine. Merck (the manufacturer of both) makes a combination vaccine that contains all four diseases in one shot, called ProQuad. The manufacturing process, ingredients, and side effects are all identical to those associated with the two separate shots. If you are going to get both shots, it makes sense to use the combo shot instead of two separate injections. As of this writing, there is a shortage of ProQuad.

Some parents choose to get the M, M, and R components in separate injections. While this does mean extra shots, exposing the body to only one virus at a time may mean fewer side effects and better vaccine effectiveness. Some doctors and researchers who suspect the MMR vaccine may play a role in autism also feel it is safer to give the three injections separately, spaced about one year apart. I can't find enough research to determine if this precaution is justified, but in theory it does make sense. However, the ingredients of each separate vaccine are almost identical (except for the specific virus in each vaccine), so separate injections expose a person to these ingredients three times instead of just once. Here is a brief look at these three separate shots. They are made by Merck and in the same manner as the MMR vaccine:

Measles vaccine (Attenuvax). The manufacturing process and ingredients for plain measles are identical to those in the full MMR vaccine except that the rubella and mumps are left out. The side effects of the single measles vaccine are identical to those listed for the full MMR vaccine, except for the rubella-associated arthritis and the mumps-associated effects (pancreas inflammation, diabetes, swollen salivary glands in the face, and testicle inflammation).

Mumps vaccine (Mumpsvax). The manufacturing process and ingredients for plain mumps are identical to those in the full MMR vaccine, except rubella and measles are left out. The side

DOES THE MMR VACCINE CAUSE AUTISM?

This debate began in 1998 when a British researcher named Dr. Wakefield published an article in *The Lancet* (see "Resources," page 257) about twelve autistic kids who had inflammatory disease in their intestines that might have been triggered by the live measles virus in the MMR vaccine. Later research showed it was the vaccine strain of measles that was infecting these kids' intestines, not a natural measles infection. The researcher never said the MMR caused the autism. He just pointed out the fact that vaccine-induced measles seemed to occur in the intestines of autistic kids and said further research should be done to investigate this possible correlation. It would take an entire book to discuss this issue completely, but here are the main points that this researcher and others have discovered over the past few years:

- Many autistic kids have a viral-induced inflammation in their intestines. The vaccine-strain measles virus is present in their intestines. Their nonautistic siblings who volunteered to be tested do not have this infection. (See "Resources," page 257.)
- Many autistic kids have evidence of the vaccine-strain measles virus in their brain and spinal fluid (obtained by spinal tap), and their siblings don't. (See "Resources," page 258.)

While these factors in no way prove that the measles component of the MMR vaccine caused these kids' autism, a few researchers, and some worried parents, believe that when com-

effects are similar to the MMR vaccine's, except that the worst neurologic side effects (encephalopathy and encephalitis) are less common. The rubella-associated arthritis doesn't seem to occur with the plain mumps vaccine.

bined with genetic predisposition and other environmental and medical factors, the measles vaccine may help trigger autism. They worry that the live measles in the vaccine may move into the intestines, cause inflammation and infection there, then spread to the brain and trigger inflammation that leads to autistic changes in the brain. Some researchers think it is possible that the mercury that used to be in other vaccines (it was never in the MMR vaccine) damaged the immune system of some kids, leaving them more susceptible to this measles virus cascade. Now that mercury is gone, this may be less of a worry.

Wakefield's work sparked a worldwide debate on this issue. Extensive investigation has been conducted, and no one has been able to prove that the MMR vaccine causes autism. Most of the doctors who worked with Wakefield have retracted the study's claims. Many epidemiological studies have found no correlation between autism and the MMR vaccine, yet some studies do claim evidence of a possible relationship. More recent studies done independently of Wakefield have duplicated his findings that viral-induced intestinal inflammatory disease in autistic kids may be linked to the vaccine-strain measles virus. See "Resources," page 255, to review all these studies.

So, who is right? We may not know with 100 percent certainty for many years. I hope someday researchers can reach a consensus that explains why some autistic children seem to have measles-related intestinal and brain inflammation and their siblings don't.

What about a possible connection between all the other vaccines and autism? I discuss that issue on page 183.

Rubella vaccine (Meruvax II). The manufacturing process and ingredients for plain rubella are identical to those in the full MMR vaccine, except measles and mumps are left out. The side effects are similar to the MMR vaccine's, except that the neurologic effects are less common. The arthritis side effect seems the same in both the full MMR and the plain rubella vaccine.

An additional note on the rubella vaccine. During pregnancy, a woman is tested to see if she has rubella immunity. If she is not immune, the health care provider will offer the rubella shot to the mom after the baby is born. This is usually done in the hospital before she goes home. Women who already suffer from arthritis or have a strong family history of rheumatoid arthritis should be aware of the potential for arthritis when they get this shot and should weigh the risk of being susceptible to rubella during future pregnancies versus the risk of arthritis side effects from the shot. (See "Chronic Arthritis," page 90.)

THE WAY I SEE IT

Although there are three diseases involved in this vaccine, parents do have the option to get each component separately, so it makes sense to consider each disease individually. Measles can be serious at any age, but it usually isn't and it's very rare. Mumps is serious mainly after childhood, and it's a little more common than measles (especially with the recent outbreak). Rubella is a completely harmless disease to children and adults alike, but it would cause more and more birth defects if allowed to escalate in our country.

While each disease is very different, the separate vaccines are quite similar. The unusual manufacturing process and potential side effects (though very rare) of each vaccine understandably give some parents pause. Given the bad press for the MMR vaccine in recent years, I'm not surprised when a family, especially one with a history of autoimmune or neurologic diseases or with one autistic child already, tells me they don't want the MMR or at least want to split it up or delay it. Since the fatality or complication rates for these childhood diseases are fairly low, I don't have much ammunition with which to try to change these parents' minds. I do point out that mumps can be serious when their kids grow up, and rubella may be an issue for their older daughters someday, and I urge them to do blood testing (see page 227) to determine the need for these shots later on. I also warn them not to share their fears with their neighbors, because if too many people avoid the MMR, we'll likely see the diseases increase significantly.

Update: In 2009 Merck decided to stop producing the separate measles, mumps, and rubella vaccines. Separating this vaccine is a prominent feature of my alternative vaccine schedule. Unfortunately, that option is no longer available to you. You'll have to decide whether your child should get the full MMR at age 1 and 5 as recommended by the CDC, or whether you should delay it or skip it altogether. My advice is to go ahead and have your child vaccinated as recommended if you feel comfortable doing so. If you have concerns about the MMR, delay it. You could safely delay the vaccine until your child enters school, since he is unlikely to come into contact with anyone who has one of these three illnesses. Once a child enters daycare or school, however, the chance of exposure increases. So I do recommend that a child get the MMR prior to daycare or school entry. Those children who do not receive the vaccine until age 4 only need one dose, as the vaccine works better the older the child is. Those who get the vaccine at age 2 or 3 may or may not need a second dose at age 5. Your doctor can do a blood test at age 5 to determine if the one dose worked well enough before you automatically proceed with the second dose. I would also recommend that the MMR be given several months away from any other vaccine. I will provide further information and updates regarding this issue at www.TheVaccineBook.com.

8

Chickenpox Disease and the Varicella Vaccine

WHAT IS CHICKENPOX?

Chickenpox is a virus that causes fever and spots all over the body. (How's that for a simple explanation?) It is easily diagnosed simply by observing the pattern of the spots. If there is any doubt, a blood test can be done to confirm the illness. It is transmitted like the common cold, and most people catch it only once. The medical term for this disease is varicella. Once a person is infected with it, the virus lives permanently within the nerves of the body. Occasionally the virus will flare up during the adult years and cause what is called shingles (the medical term is zoster). These are chickenpox-like spots that occur only in one area of the body.

IS CHICKENPOX COMMON?

No, but it used to be. Prior to vaccination (which began in the mid-1990s), we saw about 3.5 million cases each year in the

The Varicella Vaccine
American Academy of Pediatrics
2007 Recommended Vaccine Schedule

Birth	Hep B
1 month	Hep B
2 months	HIB, Pc, DTaP, Rotavirus, Polio
4 months	HIB, Pc, DTaP, Rotavirus, Polio
6 months	HIB, Pc, DTaP, Rotavirus, Hep B, Flu
1 year	MMR, **Chickenpox,** Hep A
15 months	HIB, Pc
18 months	DTaP, Polio, Hep A, Flu
2 years	Flu
3 years	Flu
4 years	Flu
5 years	DTaP, Polio, MMR, Flu, **Chickenpox**
12 years	Tdap, Meningococcal, HPV (3 doses, girls only)

United States. Since this is not a disease that gets routinely reported to the CDC by doctors, we aren't sure how common it still is. Estimates show there's been approximately a 75 percent decrease in chickenpox since vaccination began. Cases that are reported number about 50,000 each year.

IS CHICKENPOX SERIOUS?

Yes and no, but mostly no. The disease is fatal in only about 1 in every 65,000 cases. Back when it was common, it caused about fifty-five deaths each year in the United States. Now deaths are extremely rare. For example, in 2003 only two deaths were reported from chickenpox (two teens, aged twelve and eighteen).

Teens and adults who catch chickenpox usually feel much sicker than do children. Very rare complications of chickenpox (less than 1 percent of cases) include skin infections, pneumonia, arthritis, bleeding problems, kidney or liver problems, and neurologic symptoms.

Chickenpox is most serious for children or adults with compromised immune systems (such as those taking chronic steroids or suffering from any immune-related diseases).

If a pregnant woman catches chickenpox during the first half of pregnancy, it can cause birth defects. It is usually harmless in the second half of pregnancy. However, if a pregnant woman comes down with chickenpox within five days of delivery or in the first two days after the baby is born, the newborn may contract a more aggressive case of the disease, and the fatality rate for the baby would be high.

IS CHICKENPOX TREATABLE?

Yes. An antiviral medication called acyclovir (similar to an antibiotic), if started within seventy-two hours of the beginning of the rash, can make this disease less bothersome. Starting this medicine within twenty-four hours of the first spots shows the best effect. An injection of chickenpox antibodies (a medication called VZIG) can be given to people expected to suffer a severe course of the illness. If a susceptible individual gets exposed to the disease and he's never had the vaccine, the vaccine administered during the week or two after exposure may provide some protection. In most cases, however, no treatment is given and the illness just runs its course.

The chickenpox vaccine is called the varicella vaccine. The only brand used in the United States is called Varivax and is made by Merck. This vaccine has been recommended for all kids since 1995.

A version of this vaccine called Zostavax was just approved in 2007 for use in adults sixty years and older to prevent shingles (an adult flare-up of chickenpox on only one area of the body). The vaccine appears to be virtually identical to the Varivax vaccine in manufacturing and ingredients. The only difference I could find was the dosage. Zostavax gives about 25 percent more vaccine solution in the injection. The only side effect that stands out in the initial safety studies is heart trouble. Out of 3000 elderly adults who got the shot, 10 reported having a heart attack or near heart attack within 42 days. In the placebo group of 3000, only 5 reported this happening. In a larger study of 18,000 vaccinated people, there were 45 cardiac events, compared with 35 in the placebo group of 18,000. The vaccine shouldn't be given to any elderly adults with immune disorders.

WHEN IS THE VARICELLA VACCINE GIVEN?

We give the chickenpox shot at twelve months, or at any time thereafter (we don't give it earlier because live-virus vaccines like varicella and MMR don't work well before age one). A booster dose is given at age five. This booster is a brand-new recommendation as of 2007, and it should give kids longer-lasting protection. We don't yet know how long this second dose will last, but it will probably help protect kids well into the teen years.

Kids who skip this vaccine during infancy but get it when they are school age really need to get only one shot instead of two, as long as this one shot is given after age four. Some states, however, require two doses for such kids.

Teens and adults who've never had the shot need two doses spaced one to two months apart to make the vaccine work well.

HOW IS THE VARICELLA VACCINE MADE?

The virus was taken from an infected individual decades ago and placed in a culture of lung cells from human embryos. The virus used the lung cells to multiply. The viruses were then removed and placed in a culture of guinea pig embryo cells for further growth. Finally, they were put in a culture of human diploid cells (a high-tech engineered group of laboratory cells— I'm not sure what type of human tissue they originated from) to multiply even more. These viruses were then taken to Merck's laboratories.

Merck keeps the virus replicating in a different human diploid cell culture nourished with serum from a cow fetus (the liquid part of the cow fetus's blood) and removes batches of the virus to go into the vaccine. The viruses are put into a solution of saline, sugar, electrolytes, MSG, and gelatin.

The virus is whole and living when injected, so it can potentially cause chickenpox.

WHAT INGREDIENTS ARE IN THE FINAL VACCINE SOLUTION?

The varicella vaccine contains:

- The live virus
- Sucrose (sugar)
- Saline solution
- Gelatin
- MSG (like in Chinese food, but only a fraction of that amount—500 micrograms per dose)
- Potassium (an electrolyte)
- Residual components of the Merck human diploid cells, including DNA and proteins from the cells
- EDTA (a chemical used in a variety of products) in trace amounts
- Neomycin (an antibiotic used to keep the cell cultures sterile) in trace amounts
- Trace quantities of the cow fetus serum

Are any of these ingredients controversial?

- MSG has always been controversial when it comes to food. Some people are severely allergic to it, and research shows it may affect brain function (see "Resources," page 268). The amount in the vaccine is minuscule compared with the millions of micrograms a person would eat at dinner at a restaurant.
- The DNA and proteins from the human cells are an unavoidable byproduct of this particular manufacturing process. These aren't

known to be harmful, but some parents find it a little odd to inject unknown human DNA into a baby.

- Cow fetus serum. See page 192 for more information on the controversy surrounding this.
- The general use of human and animal cells to make vaccines is considered controversial by some people. See page 191 for more info.

WHAT ARE THE SIDE EFFECTS OF THE VARICELLA VACCINE?

The standard side effects (see page 180) occur at about an average rate compared with other vaccines. Some reactions unique to this vaccine are:

- A rash occurs in about 4 percent of people around two weeks after the shot. This isn't contagious.
- Flu-like symptoms (body aches and pains) may occur.

Additional reactions reported since the vaccine went on the market include:

- Bleeding problems
- Pneumonia
- Skin infections
- Severe, life-threatening rash
- Nervous system effects, including Guillain-Barré syndrome (see page 181), encephalitis (brain inflammation; see page 181), seizures, and stroke

Most of these reactions are also possible complications of the disease itself. So, both the disease and the vaccine have risks.

SHOULD YOU GIVE YOUR BABY THE VARICELLA VACCINE?

Reasons to get this vaccine

The main reason parents want their child to get this shot is that they don't want their child to have chickenpox. It can be a rough week, and, rarely, complications can occur. It can also be a very tough disease for teens and adults.

An added benefit of the shot is that if a vaccinated child does end up catching chickenpox later (the vaccine doesn't provide perfect protection), the course of the disease will be milder.

Another reason is that the illness keeps kids out of school for a week, and this can be a financial burden when both parents are working and one has to miss work to stay home with the child.

Some families have members with chronic medical conditions that would make chickenpox particularly dangerous if it spread through the family. The vaccine would be more important for them.

Parents who didn't catch chickenpox as children may feel more vulnerable to the disease and therefore may vaccinate their children to avoid catching the illness themselves.

Reasons some people choose not to get this vaccine

Perhaps the main reason some parents choose not to have their kids vaccinated for chickenpox is that they don't fear this disease. They know that chickenpox, while bothersome to go through, is usually harmless in the long run (except for the extremely rare fatality). Parents who had this illness themselves may view it as a normal rite of passage for kids.

Some parents actually *want* their kids to catch chickenpox. They may purposely get their child exposed to get the disease over with. If you've ever been invited to a "chickenpox party," you'll know what I'm referring to. Having the disease in most cases provides lifelong immunity (better immunity than the shot provides), so there is practically no worry about catching the disease as an adult. This is especially important for girls, since immunity to chickenpox during the childbearing years is useful to have.

Parents also know that if their kids do catch the disease, they can use the antiviral medication to make the illness a little easier on their child.

Additionally, some parents worry that the shot may wear off, leaving their child susceptible as an adult. The newly recommended five-year booster dose should make this less likely.

Finally, some parents may find the manufacturing process and final ingredients in this vaccine a little unusual and may avoid the shot on that basis alone.

What should parents do if their unvaccinated kids become teenagers and they haven't had chickenpox? If their kids catch the disease as teens or adults, it may be fairly severe. Well, there's hope. Kids can get a blood test to see if they were exposed to chickenpox enough to become immune, even though they did not show symptoms. If they show immunity, the parents (and kids) can rest easy. If the blood test shows they are susceptible, the family has a decision to make: to take their chances with the disease or have their kids vaccinated. See page 227 for more information on blood testing for disease immunity.

One positive note for these unvaccinated and susceptible teens and young adults: Ten years from now chickenpox will likely be as rare as measles and mumps are now. So your chance of getting sick might be much lower than it is today.

Travel considerations

The United States and Canada are virtually the only countries that vaccinate against chickenpox. So travel to any other part of the world increases an unvaccinated person's chance of catching the disease (unless they've already had it). However, since chickenpox is still fairly common in the United States, travel doesn't increase the risk enough to make this an important vaccine for international travel just yet.

Options to consider when getting this vaccine

Chickenpox is routinely given at one year and five years of age, at the same time as the MMR vaccine. Merck (the manufacturer of both) makes a combination vaccine that contains all four diseases in one shot (called ProQuad; see page 93). Parents can choose to get the MMR and chickenpox vaccines together in one shot at age one as well as in the five-year booster. While research has shown that side effects don't seem to occur more frequently when the chickenpox and MMR vaccines are given at the same time (rather than at separate visits), theoretically it makes sense that exposing the body to four diseases simultaneously may put a bigger strain on the immune system and cause more side effects. This is simply theoretical, though.

Taking vitamins A and C (see page 189 for dosage) before and after this shot is thought to be beneficial, just as it is for most shots.

THE WAY I SEE IT

Chickenpox. It used to be an everyday household word. Now it strikes fear into the heart of every parent and teacher. I'm not sure why that is. Many parents call me in a panic because it's going around the school and they don't want their kids to catch it, presumably because if they *do* catch chickenpox, they must wear a scarlet *C* on their shirt for three weeks (especially if they weren't vaccinated) while everyone around them waits for the dreadful epidemic to pass.

With most kids getting vaccinated, chickenpox is becoming less and less common. Even now I see or hear about only one or two cases each month among my patients.

However, it doesn't surprise me, given how this vaccine is made, that some parents still decide to chance the spots rather than the shot. But here's the deal: If you decide not to get the shot, you must accept the reality that your child may catch chickenpox. You can't panic if your child gets exposed. If your unvaccinated child doesn't catch chickenpox by the time he is eleven, you may want him to get the shot then if a blood test shows he is susceptible.

Since chickenpox is usually harmless, I don't worry too much when parents tell me they don't want this shot for their child. Many parents view it as an optional shot. Kids who get the shot usually grow up without the disease. Kids who don't get the shot usually either catch the disease or get the shot when they are pre-teens. The only problem with this approach is that if enough kids remain unvaccinated, the disease will continue at a certain level, making it an ongoing issue. It would be easier if every single person got the shot for the next twenty years, and we could eliminate chickenpox from the United States and then stop vaccinating for it. But I don't think this will happen because enough parents would rather let their kids get the disease over with (and have lifelong immunity) than get the shot and possibly have it wear off later. Interesting dilemma. I'm glad I'm not a public health official whose job it is to make the United States chickenpox free.

9

Hepatitis A Disease and the Hep A Vaccine

WHAT IS HEP A?

Hepatitis A is a virus that attacks the liver and causes temporary liver inflammation. Most children who get the virus don't have any symptoms at all. Teens and adults who get sick usually experience fairly severe intestinal flu symptoms that can last for a few weeks. Often jaundice (yellow skin and eyes due to liver damage) will occur in teens and adults and that's when the illness is usually diagnosed, with a blood test. Jaundice virtually never occurs in children, so hep A is rarely recognized in kids.

An infected person passes the virus in his or her stools. It is transmitted when a person comes into contact with infected stools and then ingests the virus. (Warning: If you are easily grossed out, you might want to skip the rest of this paragraph.) This most commonly occurs in day-care centers, where a care-taker's hands might get contaminated from changing the diaper of an infected infant (the baby probably doesn't even have symp-toms) and the caretaker doesn't wash his or her hands. The virus then gets into everything the caretaker touches, such as food and

The Hepatitis A Vaccine
American Academy of Pediatrics
2007 Recommended Vaccine Schedule

Birth	Hep B
1 month	Hep B
2 months	HIB, Pc, DTaP, Rotavirus, Polio
4 months	HIB, Pc, DTaP, Rotavirus, Polio
6 months	HIB, Pc, DTaP, Rotavirus, Hep B, Flu
1 year	MMR, Chickenpox, **Hep A**
15 months	HIB, Pc
18 months	DTaP, Polio, **Hep A,** Flu
2 years	Flu
3 years	Flu
4 years	Flu
5 years	DTaP, Polio, MMR, Flu, Chickenpox
12 years	Tdap, Meningococcal, HPV (3 doses, girls only)

other babies. The infection can be passed on in restaurants and homes, too. An infected person uses the bathroom (he may not know he's infected) and doesn't wash his hands. The virus then gets on any food or utensils he touches. This is how outbreaks occur.

Sometimes beaches can become contaminated with hep A by sewage runoff. This is the type of hepatitis that surfers or ocean swimmers are thought to be at risk of catching.

In developing countries the virus often infects water supplies that are contaminated through poor or nonexistent sewage treatment. Most Third World children therefore catch the disease when they are young enough not to be affected by it and grow up with lifelong immunity.

Very rarely, hep A is passed through blood transfusions or the sharing of IV drug needles.

It takes about four weeks for an exposed person to begin to feel sick. A person is most contagious during the week before symptoms begin, so community epidemics are quite easily started.

IS HEP A COMMON?

Somewhat. There are about 10,000 cases reported each year in the United States. Most cases occur in kids age five to fourteen. It is fairly rare in adults over forty. Hepatitis A occurs mainly in selected areas in the United States (Arizona, Alaska, Oregon, New Mexico, Utah, Washington, Oklahoma, South Dakota, Idaho, Nevada, and California). Other areas of the country see very little hep A.

IS HEP A SERIOUS?

It depends on how old you are. Only 30 percent of infected kids six years and under even act sick with hep A, and if they do, it's only with mild intestinal flu symptoms. Kids six to twelve years are more likely to feel sick, but their symptoms are usually mild. Teens and adults, on the other hand, usually suffer from fairly bothersome intestinal flu symptoms that can last for as long as a few weeks. Rarely, the disease can come and go for six months. People with underlying liver disease can suffer fairly severe liver damage from hep A. Thankfully, virtually all adults recover in a few weeks with no ill effects.

IS HEP A TREATABLE?

No. There is no medication that fights the hep A virus.

Hep A outbreaks

Hep A outbreaks are usually small and isolated. There are some preventive measures that can be taken for anyone exposed during an outbreak. An antibody shot (not a vaccine, but actual antibodies that kill the virus right away) called immune globulin, if given within two weeks of a person's exposure, has an 85 percent chance of preventing hep A disease. If more than fourteen days have passed since exposure, however, this antibody shot isn't effective. It can be given to infants and adults of any age. It helps contain the outbreak and prevents a widening epidemic, but since the disease is harmless in kids, most parents do not get this injection for their kids. Exposed teens and adults, on the other hand, may want this injection, since hep A can be rough for them. Immune globulin is made by filtering the antibodies out of donated human blood units. The antibodies are chemically treated and filtered to prevent transmission of any infectious diseases from the human blood donors.

In the event of an outbreak, the actual hep A vaccine can also be given to anyone two years and older if they haven't already been vaccinated. If given within two weeks of exposure to the disease, it may prevent the disease. On the other hand, since hep A is harmless to a young child, the vaccine isn't critical for children who are part of an outbreak.

WHEN IS THE HEP A VACCINE GIVEN?

Until 2006, this vaccine was not routinely given to all children. It has been available since the mid-1980s but was recommended only for kids two years and older who were living in an area with a high rate of hep A (the eleven states listed on page 111). Most other states didn't make it a part of their automatic childhood vaccine schedule back then.

Now, however, the vaccine has become part of the routine schedule in an effort to eliminate the disease from our entire country. Infants get one dose at twelve months of age, with a booster dose six to twelve months later. Anyone who gets the vaccine at an older age gets the same two shots, separated by at least six months.

HOW IS THE HEP A VACCINE MADE?

There are two brands of hep A vaccine: Vaqta, by Merck, and Havrix, by GlaxoSmithKline. Although the manufacturing process for the two brands is very similar, there is some variation in the ingredients used. These differences are discussed below.

A weakened hep A virus strain is grown and multiplied in

human cells (called human diploid fibroblasts, which are human cells modified to live in a laboratory environment). The human cells are broken up, and the intracellular solution (where the hep A virus lives) is removed, purified, and filtered. Formalin (a chemical similar to formaldehyde) is added to make sure the hep A viruses are inactivated so they don't cause infection. Aluminum is added to make the vaccine work better.

The vaccine contains whole, but inactivated, hep A virus. There's no way to become infected by the vaccine.

WHAT INGREDIENTS ARE IN THE FINAL VACCINE SOLUTION?

The vaccine contains:

- The hep A virus
- Aluminum—250 micrograms per dose
- Saline solution

Some of the ingredients in the two brands of the hep A vaccine vary slightly. Vaqta (Merck) also has the following:

- Residual proteins and DNA from the human cell line
- Traces of cow blood proteins (albumin), which are used to nourish the human cell line
- Formaldehyde
- Sodium borate (to decrease acidity)
- "Other residual chemicals at a level of 10 parts per billion" (the actual chemicals aren't listed in the PI)

Havrix (GlaxoSmithKline) adds the following to the original ingredients.

- 2-phenoxyethanol (0.5 percent of the vaccine solution), which is used as a preservative

- Amino acids (0.3 percent of the vaccine solution), which are used to nourish the human cells
- Polysorbate 20 (25 micrograms)
- Formalin
- Residual proteins from the human cells
- Neomycin (extremely minute traces), an antibiotic used to keep the cell culture sterile

Are any of these ingredients controversial?

- Aluminum (see pages 193 to 206)
- Formaldehyde (see page 209)
- Cow blood proteins in the Vaqta brand (see page 191)
- Human cell proteins in the Havrix brand (see page 191)
- 2-phenoxyethanol and polysorbate 20 in the Havrix brand (see pages 209 and 210)

WHAT ARE THE SIDE EFFECTS OF THE HEP A VACCINE?

Standard side effects are similar to those found with other vaccines, except that pain, swelling, and redness at the injection site are more common than with most shots. Headache and loss of appetite are a bit more common, too.

In the initial safety trials of seven hundred infants using the Vaqta brand, seizures occurred in 1 percent of infants aged twelve to twenty-three months. Other vaccines were also given during this study period, so it isn't known which vaccine, if any, was associated with the seizures. Seizures were much less common when the hep A vaccine was given to kids two years and older. This may be why the vaccine previously wasn't recommended until age two. Now, however, experts feel the seizure risk is small enough for the vaccine to be given at twelve months.

Very rarely, Guillain-Barré syndrome, encephalitis (brain inflammation), encephalopathy (brain dysfunction), nerve problems, and multiple sclerosis have been reported. See page 181 for more discussion on these serious side effects.

SHOULD YOU GIVE YOUR BABY THIS VACCINE?

Reasons to get this vaccine

The main benefit that comes from young children getting this vaccine in areas of the country that have hep A is that all kids in that area will have protection in the event of an outbreak.

Vaccinating young children will also help protect the adults around them, for whom hep A infection can be more serious.

The vaccine also offers some protection to these kids as they grow up, when hep A would be more serious. The disease can be very long and tough to go through for teenagers or adults. Time off from work or school can be a burden.

Having the shot as a child also gives protection during travel to underdeveloped countries, where hep A is more common (see "Travel Considerations," next page).

People with chronic liver diseases should get the vaccine, since hep A disease is particularly serious for them.

Reasons some people choose not to get this vaccine

Some parents consider vaccines for their children only for diseases that are somewhat severe. Since hep A is virtually harmless for children, some parents decline it.

The chemical ingredients, human cells, and cow blood proteins may concern some parents.

Even in the event of an outbreak, some parents would prefer to just let their kids go through this mild disease.

Parents who don't live in a hep A state may consider the vaccine less important.

To decrease the risk of seizures, some parents may delay this vaccine until after age two.

Travel considerations

Hepatitis A is very common in underdeveloped countries. Virtually all kids living there get hep A. They get lifetime immunity, and therefore don't have to worry about the disease as an adult. However, U.S. citizens who don't typically get hep A as children could easily catch hep A from the water or food in a Third World country. The person probably wouldn't even feel sick until he got back to the States, but it's still no fun if you are laid up in bed for weeks.

Places that typically don't have hep A disease are Western Europe, Scandinavia, Australia, New Zealand, Japan, and Canada, so the vaccine isn't needed for travel there. Travel to most other areas of the world could pose a risk. Most people don't have time to get both doses of the shot before they travel (unless they plan about seven months ahead), but even one shot gives some protection. See www.cdc.gov/travel/diseases.htm for up-to-date information on hep A worldwide.

Options to consider when getting this vaccine

Since the shot contains aluminum, it may be prudent to get it separately from other aluminum shots.

There is a vaccine called Twinrix (GlaxoSmithKline) that combines the hep A (Havrix brand, page 114) and hep B (Engerix-B brand, page 54) vaccines in one shot. This is only for people eighteen years and older, so it's not a decision you would make for a child. However, any of you adults who feel you need both hep A and hep B protection (for example, if you plan to go to a Third World country and get a tattoo, eat questionable food from a street vendor, and have unprotected sex with a stranger), ask your doctor about using this one shot instead of the separate vaccines. The manufacturing and ingredients are virtually identical to the separate Havrix and Engerix-B vaccines—they're just combined together in one injection.

THE WAY I SEE IT

Since this is a benign disease in young children, I did not used to give the vaccine routinely in my office when it wasn't required. I've seen only a few cases of hep A, during a local outbreak from a restaurant a few years ago. Now that the hep A vaccine is universally recommended, more doctors give it. I'm still on the fence. On the one hand, hep A can be a very tough virus for teens and adults. Universal use of this vaccine in children may eventually eliminate the disease from the United States. On the other hand, it's such a mild disease in children, why vaccinate for it? But if a significant number of kids skip this vaccine, we'll never rid our population of the disease. It will continue to be a risk for adults. I think it makes sense to wait until a child is at least two years old to give this shot in order to lower the risk of a seizure side effect.

10

Influenza Disease and the Flu Vaccine

WHAT IS THE FLU?

The flu, or influenza, is a virus that hits the United States every year in the late fall and winter. There are different strains of the flu virus around the world, and usually a different strain predominates every year. The flu is transmitted like the common cold, and symptoms include fever, headache, body ache, sore throat, vomiting, diarrhea, stuffy nose, runny nose, cough, and so forth. You name it, the flu can probably cause it. It is usually diagnosed by observation of the various symptoms. There is a nasal swab test that can confirm whether or not a person's illness is the actual flu, but most doctors don't bother with this, since the disease isn't usually treated, anyway.

What about the avian flu (bird flu)? This dreaded strain of the flu is almost identical to the common human flu, but it mainly infects birds and usually leaves people alone. When it infects domesticated birds like chicken, ducks, and turkey, it can be particularly deadly. Very rarely, humans have become infected after contact with contaminated birds or poultry. While the bird flu

The Flu Vaccine
American Academy of Pediatrics
2007 Recommended Vaccine Schedule

Birth	Hep B
1 month	Hep B
2 months	HIB, Pc, DTaP, Rotavirus, Polio
4 months	HIB, Pc, DTaP, Rotavirus, Polio
6 months	HIB, Pc, DTaP, Rotavirus, Hep B, **Flu**
1 year	MMR, Chickenpox, Hep A
15 months	HIB, Pc
18 months	DTaP, Polio, Hep A, **Flu**
2 years	**Flu**
3 years	**Flu**
4 years	**Flu**
5 years	DTaP, Polio, MMR, **Flu**, Chickenpox
12 years	Tdap, Meningococcal, HPV (3 doses, girls only)

can be very serious for people, it is not yet thought to be transmitted from person to person. Large human outbreaks are therefore unlikely, and an avian flu vaccine is not being mass-produced as of yet. Sanofi Pasteur has developed the vaccine, and the government is holding it ready in case an epidemic does occur.

IS THE FLU COMMON?

Yes, very. It's by far the most common illness that we have a vaccine for. There are millions of cases of the flu each year. It's funny, though. Every year I hear on the news that this coming flu season is supposed to be "the worst flu season ever!" But as far as I can tell, almost every flu season has been about the same since I became a doctor. One of these years the doomsayers may be right.

IS THE FLU SERIOUS?

Mostly no, but sometimes yes. Virtually all cases of the flu pass without consequence. However, there is an average of 100,000 hospitalizations each year because of complications from the flu. Most involve elderly people.

There is a misconception about how serious the flu is in infants and children. This is because the most common source of flu data comes from the *Morbidity and Mortality Weekly Report (MMWR)* database. This is what most doctors review when they investigate flu data for any given year so they'll know how to educate their patients about the risks of the flu. The *MMWR* reports deaths from the flu and from pneumonia all in the same group. So most doctors (and regular people, too) can't easily look up how many people died from just the flu in a given year. In addition, the

MMWR doesn't tell us how many infants and young children die compared with the number of elderly adults. All the *MMWR* does tell us is that over the past several years, about 36,000 people have died annually from the flu and pneumonia. This is the statistic most commonly referred to when people talk about the flu. Most informational materials that promote the flu vaccine cite this statistic from the *MMWR,* giving the false impression that 36,000 people actually die from the flu every year. In reality, this is the number of deaths from the flu and pneumonia combined. I was reading an Associated Press news release from May 1, 2006, about a new flu vaccine, and sure enough, there it was: "Each winter, flu kills 36,000 Americans, most of them elderly." No wonder people panic over the flu. Other press releases even go so far as to say, "36,000 people die every year from the flu, most of them infants and the elderly." Such statements give worried parents the false impression that thousands, if not tens of thousands, of infants are killed each year by the flu.

What is the *actual* number of flu fatalities every year? Relatively few. How do I know this? Because the National Center for Health Statistics, a lesser-known database that doctors don't commonly read, does collect data on all causes of death in the United States. This center, along with the American Lung Association, published a paper in 2004 (see "Resources," page 267) that detailed the number of deaths from the flu alone in various age groups over the past twenty-five years. They found that there had been fewer than twenty deaths reported each year in each of the following age groups:

- Infants under 1 year
- Kids ages 1 to 4 years
- Kids ages 5 to 14 years
- Young adults ages 15 to 24 years
- Adults ages 25 to 34 years

This adds up to only about 100 deaths reportedly caused by the actual flu virus, or complications thereof, each year in children and young adults combined. The same paper says the total number of deaths from the flu each year in the United States averages about 1500. Over 90 percent of these deaths are in people age sixty-five and older.

One recent study gives us another useful look at how serious the flu is, or isn't (see "Resources," page 267). The 2003–2004 flu season was particularly bad, with more reported infections and fatalities than usual. But when all was said and done, there were a total of 153 deaths in children seventeen years and younger in the forty states that were studied. If we included all fifty states, we could guess there were at most 200 deaths in children that year. So, even in a worse-than-usual flu season four years ago, the total childhood fatalities came nowhere close to the thousands that we are led to believe.

One group of people who are at an increased risk of having a severe case of the flu are those with chronic heart, lung, or immune system diseases. Flu prevention is particularly important for them and their family members.

To summarize, the flu seems to be rarely serious in healthy infants, children, and young adults. Vaccinating infants and young children, however, does help prevent the spread of the flu to the elderly and those with chronic medical conditions.

IS THE FLU TREATABLE?

Yes. Antiviral medications, if started within forty-eight hours of the first symptoms, can make the flu milder. But because people usually don't seek medical care for the flu in the first two days of illness, most don't receive these meds and the flu must run its course. These meds are approved for infants one year and older.

WHEN IS THE FLU VACCINE GIVEN?

The flu vaccine is officially recommended for all kids between six months and five years of age every year during flu season. It is also recommended for children and adults at any age with asthma or other lung diseases, heart disease, diabetes, or immune system problems, and for all adults over sixty-five.

Healthy children and adults can get a flu vaccine at any age, even if they don't fall into a recommended category.

The first year a flu vaccine is given to kids eight years and younger, two doses (one month apart for the injection, and two months apart for the nasal spray) are needed to make the vaccine work well. In subsequent years, only one dose is needed. Kids nine and older and adults don't need two doses their first time.

The flu vaccine is given each year beginning in October, but you can get it anytime during the the late fall and winter months.

So, all babies who are six months to twenty-three months of age get one flu vaccine in October, and one in November (December if using the nasal spray). The next year, they get only one shot, in October. After that, they get a flu shot yearly in October through age five. Any child with chronic lung, heart, or immune system diseases should continue to get one shot each year after that.

The following groups of people *should not* get a flu shot, according to the product inserts:

- People who are allergic to eggs
- People who have had Guillain-Barré syndrome

In addition, the following people *should not* get the live-virus nasal spray vaccine:

- Kids under age seventeen who have a medical condition that requires them to routinely take aspirin. When aspirin is mixed with the flu (even the live-virus vaccine in the nasal spray), a life-threatening reaction called Reye's syndrome can result.
- People with chronic lung, heart, or immune system disease. The killed injected vaccine is safer for them.

HOW IS THE FLU VACCINE MADE?

There are two types of flu vaccine—a live-virus nasal spray (which can cause a flu infection) and a killed-virus injection (which cannot cause a flu infection, because the viruses are killed and split). Each year different strains are used in the vaccine to cover the predicted strains for the coming year.

Most infants, young children, and the elderly get the injection. The nasal spray was initially approved only for people age five years through fifty years, but a new version of the FluMist brand (see below), referred to as CAIV-T, is due out in 2007, and it is expected to be approved for children as young as 12 months of age. Early studies are showing that the nasal spray works 50 percent better than the injected flu shot. If it is approved, the spray may, or may not become the preferred vaccine for infants and children. We'll know more over the next couple years.

Not all brands of injected flu vaccine are approved yet for infants. In the 2006–2007 flu season, Fluzone was the only one approved starting at six months of age. Fluvirin is approved for people four years and older, and Fluarix and FluLaval are approved for those eighteen years and older. Manufacturers of flu vaccines vary from year to year. At some point a particular maker might have problems with the manufacturing process and not be able to release its vaccine in a given year. The following were the makers for the 2005–2006 and 2006–2007 winter flu seasons, and they are expected to continue in subsequent years. Other makers may exist in the future. Furthermore, production techniques may change, so the following descriptions apply only for the next few years. I will keep you updated on future flu vaccines at www.TheVaccineBook.com.

Killed-virus injection

All four brands of the injected flu vaccine used in recent years are made by the same basic process. Several strains of the flu virus are grown in chicken eggs with chicken embryos inside. The viruses are removed from the eggs, inactivated, and split open, using several chemicals. The virus particles are put into a saline solution.

The chemicals used to kill the viruses vary in the four brands.

Fluarix (GlaxoSmithKline). This brand uses sodium deoxycholate, octoxynol, and formaldehyde to inactivate the flu viruses. Mercury is also used, but most of it is filtered out.

Fluzone (Sanofi Pasteur). This brand uses formaldehyde and octoxynol for viral inactivation. Gelatin is also added to make it more stable. Mercury is added to the large ten-dose vial as a preservative. No mercury is used in the preservative-free single doses.

FluLaval (ID Biomedical Corp. of Quebec, distributed by GlaxoSmithKline). U.V. light, formaldehyde, and sodium deoxycholate are used to kill the viruses. Mercury is added as a preservative.

Fluvirin (Chiron). Fluvirin uses betapropiolactone to kill the viruses, then nonylphenol ethoxylate for further purification. Mercury is also used, then mostly filtered out.

Live-virus nasal spray

The brand name is FluMist (MedImmune). A master donor virus, or MDV (a flu virus from years ago), is grown in chick kidney cells. Genetic techniques stimulate the MDV to display some characteristics of the modern flu strains that are expected to be prevalent for that year. An antibiotic is added to prevent contaminant growth. These genetically altered viruses are then put into chicken eggs, where they multiply. The fluid from inside the eggs (which contains the flu virus) is then removed, purified, and mixed with sucrose (a sugar), potassium, and MSG. This solution is put in a nasal spray dispenser. The live virus is actually intended to multiply within the lining of the nose and throat, cause a low-grade infection, and thus stimulate immunity to the various flu strains.

For about three weeks after the vaccine is given, a person is considered slightly contagious with this live virus. Close contact with anyone who suffers from an immune-suppressing medical condition should be avoided for those three weeks.

What about the new infant form of FluMist due out in 2007? I don't know exactly how this newer infant version is made or what the ingredients are, but it is likely to be very similar to the current FluMist. I will post an update on www.TheVaccineBook.com when this information becomes available.

WHAT INGREDIENTS ARE IN THE FINAL VACCINE SOLUTION?

The Fluarix brand (killed injected vaccine) contains:

- Killed and split virus particles
- Saline solution
- Octoxynol

- Alpha-tocopheryl hydrogen succinate (this complicated word is actually just vitamin E)
- Polysorbate 80
- Mercury, used during manufacturing, then filtered out (the residual is less than 1 microgram)
- Hydrocortisone
- Gentamicin (an antibiotic)
- Formaldehyde
- Egg proteins
- Sodium deoxycholate

The Fluzone brand (killed injected vaccine) contains:

- The killed and split virus particles
- Saline solution
- Gelatin
- Egg proteins
- Formaldehyde and octoxynol. The product insert does not say how much, if any, is left over in the final product. All other vaccines that use these chemicals during manufacturing have a residual amount left over and listed in the final ingredients. I would think there would be some residual here, too.
- Mercury. The large 10-dose vial has 25 micrograms per dose, but the single-dose vials don't have any mercury.

The Fluzone brand is unique in that it provides four different types of vaccine solutions:

- A half-size single-dose prefilled syringe (mercury free) for infants age six to thirty-five months. This provides infants with only half the dose that is given to older kids and adults. Other manufacturers don't provide this option.
- A full-size single-dose vial (mercury free) for thirty-six months and older
- A full-size single-dose prefilled syringe (mercury free) for thirty-six months and older

- A large 10-dose vial containing 25 micrograms of mercury per dose for thirty-six months and older

From 2005 through 2007, Sanofi Pasteur devoted most of its manufacturing to the large ten-dose vials (with mercury) and the half-size single-dose infant prefilled syringe (mercury free). They made only a limited supply of the mercury-free single-dose vials and syringes for ages thirty-six months and older. This means that for now, most children and adults will get mercury.

The FluLaval brand (killed injected vaccine) contains:

- The killed and split virus particles
- Saline
- Mercury—the full 25 micrograms is present in each dose.
- Residual egg proteins
- Sodium deoxycholate
- Formaldehyde
- No antibiotics are used in this vaccine.

The Fluvirin brand (killed injected vaccine) contains:

- The killed and split virus particles
- Saline
- Mercury—trace amount
- Polymyxin, neomycin (both antibiotics), and betapropiolactone. These are filtered out during the manufacturing process to a level that is undetectable by current techniques.
- The product insert doesn't reveal whether or not egg proteins remain in the final vaccine solution. I suspect there are some there, since they are left over in the other brands.

The FluMist brand (live nasal spray) contains:

- The live viruses
- Fluid and proteins from the eggs

- MSG (0.45 mg)
- Potassium
- Sucrose
- Gentamicin (an antibiotic), in almost undetectable amounts

Are any of these ingredients controversial?

- The mercury in the large Fluzone and FluLaval bottles is controversial. The trace amounts in the Fluvirin and Fluarix are probably harmless.
- Formaldehyde is a toxic chemical, but the small amount here is probably harmless. See page 209 for more information.
- MSG is probably harmless in these small amounts. See page 209 for more information.
- Octoxynol, polysorbate 80, and sodium deoxycholate are all chemicals that are generally regarded as safe. See pages 209 and 211 for more information on all these chemicals.

WHAT ARE THE SIDE EFFECTS OF THE FLU VACCINE?

Any typical flu symptom can occur after the vaccine. These are fairly common with the nasal spray, where about two-thirds of people reported one or more flu symptoms within a week of the vaccine.

For the injected vaccine, flu symptoms are most common with the first injection, and less common in subsequent years.

Allergic reactions have been reported, probably due to an egg allergy.

More serious side effects include Guillain-Barré syndrome, a paralyzing condition (see page 181), which is reported in twenty to forty people every year after getting a flu vaccine. It has not been proven that the vaccine causes this reaction, since GBS also occurs in people who haven't had any recent vaccines. People with a previous history of GBS are cautioned not to get a flu vaccine.

Other neurologic reactions, such as encephalopathy (see page 181), facial and arm paralysis, and visual problems, have been reported rarely.

SHOULD YOU GIVE YOUR BABY THE FLU VACCINE?

Reasons to get this vaccine

High-risk groups (the elderly and those with chronic medical problems) benefit most from the vaccine, since catching the flu is more likely to cause severe disease and possibly death in these people. Infants in the first two years of life are also at slightly higher risk than older kids and healthy adults.

Healthy people who live with someone in a high-risk group are often vaccinated so the high-risk family member is less likely to catch the disease.

People who have suffered a difficult course of the flu in the past often get the flu vaccine to help them avoid this.

If the primary wage earner in the family catches the flu and has to miss work for several days, this can create a financial burden. If a child has two working parents, one will have to miss work if the child catches the flu.

Even though the flu is rarely fatal in children, it can create complications that require hospitalization. Getting a flu shot every year decreases this chance.

Side effects other than flu-like symptoms are fairly minimal.

Research has shown that preventing the flu decreases the chance of ear infections. This may be a good reason to get the shot for kids with recurrent ear infections.

Reasons some people choose not to get this vaccine

Some parents are reluctant to give their young babies a flu shot because of the high incidence of flu-like symptoms.

Breastfeeding mothers who stay at home typically view their babies as less susceptible to catching illnesses like the flu. They are right.

The number of infant deaths from the flu each year is very low. While these deaths are tragic, some parents view the risk as very low.

If the mercury-free vaccine isn't available for an infant, some parents may decline it for that year.

The flu shot has more chemicals than most shots. This may worry some parents.

The flu is less likely to cause hospitalization in children over age two. Some parents don't feel it's worth getting a shot every year beyond toddlerhood.

Parents know they can treat their kids with an antiviral medication if they do catch the flu, so they may feel safer about the disease.

Travel considerations

The flu is just as common in the United States as in other parts of the world. While airplane travel during the flu season may pose a slight risk, if you don't typically get a flu shot each year, travel shouldn't necessarily prompt you to get one. Internationally, the flu season is not confined to the fall and winter. In tropical regions, the flu can be found year-round. In temperate regions of the Southern Hemisphere, the flu season is the opposite of when it is in the Northern Hemisphere—it goes from April through September. Tourists traveling in a large group are especially at risk. People who get the flu shot in the winter are covered for travel the following spring and summer.

Options to consider when getting this vaccine

The killed-virus injectable vaccine seems to create side effects less often than the live-virus nasal spray. Even though it is a shot, it may be preferable. On the other hand, the nasal vaccine is more effective. Take your pick.

Try to get the flu shot without mercury—especially infants and pregnant women. Any flu shot that is taken out of a large ten-dose vial probably has mercury. Any single-dose vial shot doesn't (except for a tiny trace amount in two of the brands).

More and more states have passed laws banning mercury in vaccines for children. However, when the supply of mercury-free flu vaccine ran out during the 2006–2007 flu season, this ban was lifted, allowing doctors to use mercury-containing flu vaccine for infants and children who still needed a flu shot. Hopefully in the near future, manufacturing priorities will change and companies that make mercury-free flu vaccine will focus their efforts in that department. Then everyone will be able to go mercury free.

The ages of your children determine the brands you can choose from. For kids six months through age three, the Fluzone shot is your only option. The nasal spray may soon become available for one-year-olds and up. Kids four years and older can choose either Fluzone or Fluvirin shots. The nasal spray is a choice by age five years. Fluarix and FluLaval are approved for adults only, as are all the other brands.

THE WAY I SEE IT

The most important issue regarding the flu shot is to make sure you don't get one with the full mercury dose. One brand that has the full mercury dose is also the brand that makes a completely mercury-free option. The two other brands do contain a trace of mercury, but this is negligible. Even though no one has proven that mercury is definitely harmful in a shot, it just makes good sense not to get it if you have a choice.

It's too early to tell whether or not the nasal spray will become the preferred method for infants, children, and adults. It's nice to avoid an injection, but the higher chance of side effects may be quite bothersome to babies. Look for updates on this at www.TheVaccineBook.com.

Like every other doctor, I see cases of the flu every day in my office during flu season. There's no doubt that it is a very common and uncomfortable disease to go through, but I feel that the potential severity of the flu for infants and children has been hyped by the media. The actual number of fatalities in this age group every year is extremely small. Combine this with the high rate of side effects and the unusual chemical additives in the shot, and it's no wonder some parents shy away from making this a routine vaccine for their kids.

So, have your kids get the flu shot if you don't want them to go through a tough week, or if they or someone in your household is at high risk. But the flu isn't a disease you should live in fear of. Don't panic just because you hear on the news, "This will be the worst flu season *ever!*"

The Pandemic H1N1 Flu Virus, or "Swine Flu"
Check www.TheVaccineBook.com for timely and important information on swine flu disease and the swine flu vaccine.

11

Meningococcal Disease and the Meningococcal Vaccine

WHAT IS MENINGOCOCCAL DISEASE?

The *Meningococcus* bacterium causes an infection that runs through the bloodstream to various body organs and can spread to the brain and cause meningitis. It is transmitted like the common cold. It has a very rapid onset. Symptoms begin with simple aches and fever but can progress to full symptoms of meningitis (high fever, severe headache, neck stiffness, and vomiting) within twenty-four hours. A unique feature of meningococcal (pronounced men-in-joe-*kock*-al) disease is its characteristic rash—red pinpoint dots (they look like dots made from a fine-tipped red pen, and they don't blanch or disappear when the skin is pulled tight around them) that progress to become larger purple splotches all over the body. Diagnosis is made through blood testing and/or a spinal tap.

The Meningococcal Vaccine
American Academy of Pediatrics
2007 Recommended Vaccine Schedule

Birth	Hep B
1 month	Hep B
2 months	HIB, Pc, DTaP, Rotavirus, Polio
4 months	HIB, Pc, DTaP, Rotavirus, Polio
6 months	HIB, Pc, DTaP, Rotavirus, Hep B, Flu
1 year	MMR, Chickenpox, Hep A
15 months	HIB, Pc
18 months	DTaP, Polio, Hep A, Flu
2 years	Flu
3 years	Flu
4 years	Flu
5 years	DTaP, Polio, MMR, Flu, Chickenpox
12 years	Tdap, **Meningococcal**,* HPV (3 doses, girls only)

Note: Approval for use in children as young as age two is pending.

IS MENINGOCOCCAL DISEASE COMMON?

There are about 3000 cases each year in the United States. Most cases occur in infants six months to two years of age. Some occur in college freshmen living in close quarters and in military personnel living in barracks. This type of meningitis is commonly thought of as "dormitory meningitis."

IS MENINGOCOCCAL DISEASE SERIOUS?

Yes, it is extremely serious. This is probably the single most serious and potentially deadly of all vaccine-preventable diseases. Out of the 3000 yearly cases, about 10 percent are fatal. Even more concerning is that for teens and college-age kids, about 20 percent of cases are fatal. Out of approximately 250 teen and college-age cases each year in the United States, about fifty are fatal.

Even when the disease is not fatal, aggressive medical care in an ICU for weeks is usually required. This is because the disease attacks many organs in the body, which then shut down until the body responds to antibiotics. About 15 percent of survivors of this disease have some sort of permanent disability, such as nerve damage, hearing loss, or (very rarely) loss of a limb from overwhelming infection.

IS MENINGOCOCCAL DISEASE TREATABLE?

Yes. Antibiotics are given intravenously for about a week. However, because the disease has such a rapid onset and is sometimes so damaging to internal organs, antibiotics aren't always enough once the disease has been contracted. People who are exposed to someone with meningococcal disease should take oral antibiotics right away to prevent the disease.

WHEN IS THE MENINGOCOCCAL VACCINE GIVEN?

This is a brand-new vaccine—it came into widespread use in 2005. It is given in one dose at age eleven or twelve. It is recommended that any high school kids who missed that dose get vaccinated at the first opportunity. The shot is given to all college freshmen who will be living in dormitories (the highest-risk population among college students) if they haven't received it before. While it is not officially recommended for other college-age groups, it can be given if desired.

The initial demand for this vaccine was higher than estimated, and we've run into a slight shortage. The manufacturer (Sanofi Pasteur) is opening a new facility in 2008 that should be able to meet the demand. In the meantime, the CDC has asked that the vaccine be reserved for the highest-risk groups: kids entering high school, college students living in dorms, and military recruits. Once the supply increases, we will once again begin vaccinating at the target age of eleven or twelve.

Interestingly, this disease is most common in infants less than two years old. So, why don't we vaccinate babies? As of this writing, the vaccine hasn't been approved yet for younger kids. We are not sure how well the shot will work or if the side effects will be tolerated by them. This vaccine is currently being studied in kids as young as two years of age, and the FDA is reviewing the data on its safety and effectiveness. It's possible we may begin giving it to two-year-olds as early as 2008 and eventually younger infants within the next few years. For right now, only adolescents are being targeted for protection.

The only brand of this vaccine in the United States is Menactra, by Sanofi Pasteur. The same manufacturer also makes Menomune, an older form of this vaccine. This older version was used on an optional basis and to control outbreaks, but since immunity lasted only a few years, it was never recommended for universal use in teens. The newer Menactra gives long-lasting immunity.

HOW IS THE MENINGOCOCCAL VACCINE MADE?

The bacteria (probably originally taken from an infected person) are maintained in petri dishes in a laboratory. Batches of the bacteria are broken up, and the sugars that cover the outer shell of the germs are filtered out. Diptheria bacteria are also grown separately. The toxin produced by the diphtheria is filtered out and combined with the *Meningococcus* sugars. These paired components are then added to a saline solution. Combining the germ's sugars with the diphtheria toxin helps the vaccine work better. This is classified as a polysaccharide conjugate vaccine, just like the HIB and Pc vaccines. There is no way to get the infection from this vaccine.

WHAT INGREDIENTS ARE IN THE FINAL VACCINE SOLUTION?

The Menactra brand contains only the following (no other chemicals are present):

- Diphtheria toxin/*Meningococcus* sugar pairs
- Saline solution

Are any of these ingredients controversial?

No, unless you are afraid of salt water. This is one of the most simple and pure vaccines available.

WHAT ARE THE SIDE EFFECTS OF
THE MENINGOCOCCAL VACCINE?

The standard reactions (fever, pain, aches; see page 180) occur more frequently with this vaccine than with most others. About 40 percent of people experience a headache or fatigue, and 20 percent feel flu-like symptoms or have joint aches. About 1 percent of people have these effects severely enough to require bed rest.

The most likely reason for these higher side effect percentages is that vaccines typically cause more reactions in teens and adults than in children. Any vaccine studies in teens and adults are going to create more side effects. So the reactions probably aren't because of the particular vaccine, but rather simply because of the targeted age group.

Since this is a new vaccine, we don't know all of the side effects that might occur with widespread use in the general population. There is one, however, that has shown up right away: Guillain-Barré syndrome (see page 181). This severe and potentially paralyzing reaction was reported six times in the first several months that this vaccine was on the market in 2005. These cases were published in various journals, and a summary is available on the *Morbidity and Mortality Weekly Report*'s Web site, www.cdc.gov/mmwr. The reactions occurred two to four weeks after the vaccine was received. Some patients still had residual weakness in parts of their bodies several months later. About 2.5 million doses of the vaccine had been distributed in the United States by this time, though it isn't known how many of these doses had actually been administered.

As of late 2007, 19 cases of GBS have been reported to the Centers for Disease Control after this vaccine was received. All reactions occurred among adolescents. Remember, this reaction isn't unique to the meningococcal vaccine. There are twenty to forty cases of GBS reported each year after the flu vaccine, as well as after several other vaccines.

There are many different causes of GBS, and researchers feel the number of reported cases is about what would be expected in our population of teens during this time period, anyway. Right now it hasn't been proven that the vaccine is responsible for this reaction, but this issue will continue to be researched. In the next few years, we will probably be able to determine exactly how the yearly number of GBS reactions compares with the actual number of doses given and come up with a percentage risk. Given what we've seen so far, I would estimate this risk to be somewhere between 1 in 100,000 and 1 in 1 million doses.

SHOULD YOU GIVE YOUR CHILD THIS VACCINE?

Reasons to get this vaccine

Obviously, meningitis is devastating. Getting the shot during the early teen years protects a child through high school and college.

Although this is a fairly rare disease, the chance that a college freshman in a dorm could catch it is something to consider. There are about 250 teen and college-age cases each year.

The ingredients are among the purest and simplest of all vaccines.

Reasons some people choose not to get this vaccine

Probably the main reason some parents choose not to get this vaccine is the rare possibility of GBS. Although it hasn't been proven that this reaction is caused by the vaccine, the slight possibility naturally concerns some parents.

The fact that the standard side effects are more common with this shot than with most others may worry some parents.

The disease itself isn't very common, so some parents may not worry too much about their kids catching it.

Some parents elect to delay this shot until their child actually goes to college, since college freshmen in dorms are the most commonly affected group (outside of infancy, that is).

As with any new vaccine, some parents may be more cautious until several years of use have gone by.

Travel considerations

This disease isn't more common in most other countries, so this isn't a vaccine to get just for travel purposes. The one exception to this is "the meningitis belt" in Africa. The countries that border the southern edge of the Sahara Desert have a high rate of meningococcal disease between December and June.

Precautions to consider when getting this vaccine

Obviously, anyone who has had GBS before should be cautious. This vaccine would be fairly risky for them. Amazingly, one of the GBS cases following this vaccine had also had GBS reactions at age two and five after childhood vaccines. You might think the family would have stopped vaccinating by now. Anyone with any significant neurologic disease should weigh the risks versus the benefits. This vaccine has not caused any problems with seizures to date, so it may not be a concern for children with seizure disorders.

THE WAY I SEE IT

No one can argue that meningococcal disease isn't a horrible thing to see, much less to actually catch. Fortunately, it is somewhat rare. I saw one case during my medical training, and I haven't seen it since. While this vaccine is an important step in eliminating or at least minimizing the disease among our nation's teens, there is a potential risk of GBS reaction. This concern may cause a slight snag in vaccination rates for this disease. If experts can determine that the risk of GBS is negligible, the shot will likely become more widely accepted.

It appears likely that this vaccine will soon be approved for kids as young as two years old. If the safety profile pans out for this younger crowd, this will become a very important vaccine, since this disease is more common in younger children.

An investigational new combination of HIB and meningococcal vaccines (a different formulation from the Menactra brand) is currently undergoing safety trials with GlaxoSmithKline for use at 2 months, 4 months, and 6 months of age. If approved, this vaccine will provide much-needed protection during infancy, when meningococcal disease is most common. Details on its production, ingredients, and expected release date are not yet available, but I will post updates at www.TheVaccineBook.com as more information comes my way.

12

Human Papillomavirus Disease and the HPV Vaccine

WHAT IS HPV?

HPV is a virus that causes genital warts. It is transmitted through unprotected sex, specifically genital contact. HPV also causes cervical cancer. In women, this virus can live within the vaginal area but not cause visible warts. Therefore, most women who carry this virus don't know they have it until they get a Pap smear. They will pass it on to most sexual partners when condoms aren't used. Men may carry this virus on their penis but not notice the warts.

IS HPV COMMON?

Most sexually active women carry this virus by the time they are in their early twenties, and most men will have come into contact with it by then and perhaps carry it as well. HPV is the most common sexually transmitted disease in the United States—an estimated twenty million people become infected with HPV each year.

The HPV Vaccine
American Academy of Pediatrics
2007 Recommended Vaccine Schedule

Birth	Hep B
1 month	Hep B
2 months	HIB, Pc, DTaP, Rotavirus, Polio
4 months	HIB, Pc, DTaP, Rotavirus, Polio
6 months	HIB, Pc, DTaP, Rotavirus, Hep B, Flu
1 year	MMR, Chickenpox, Hep A
15 months	HIB, Pc
18 months	DTaP, Polio, Hep A, Flu
2 years	Flu
3 years	Flu
4 years	Flu
5 years	DTaP, Polio, MMR, Flu, Chickenpox
12 years	Tdap, Meningococcal, **HPV** (3 doses, girls only)

IS HPV SERIOUS?

There are various strains of HPV. Some strains cause only genital warts, which often resolve by themselves without treatment. Occasionally the warts become extremely large and disfiguring.

Some strains of HPV cause cervical cancer. All cancer is very serious, but fortunately cervical cancer is usually detected early by a Pap smear, and a partial resection of the cervix provides a cure. In the United States, there are about 10,000 cases and 3500 deaths from cervical cancer each year.

IS HPV TREATABLE?

Yes. Warts can be removed in a variety of ways, including topical gels, freezing, and laser removal. None of these treatments is pleasant. Cervical cancer is usually cured in its early stages with surgical removal of a small portion of the cervix, so further treatment is often unnecessary. Chemotherapy is used for advanced cases of cervical cancer.

WHEN IS THE HPV VACCINE GIVEN?

The HPV vaccine three-shot series is started at age eleven or twelve, before sexual activity begins. The second dose is given two months after the first, and the third dose is six months after the first dose. The vaccine can be given to any woman aged nine to twenty-six years. It is not currently approved for use in boys.

Two companies have developed HPV vaccines:

Gardasil (Merck). This brand protects against the two most common strains of genital wart–causing HPV and the two main strains of cervical cancer–causing HPV. It was approved in 2006.

Cervarix (GlaxoSmithKline). Cervarix protects against the two cancer strains only. Approval is pending but is expected in late 2007 or early 2008.

You should be aware that the HPV vaccine protects against only the most common HPV strains, not *all* the strains. The two cancer-causing HPV strains covered by the vaccine account for only about 70 percent of cervical cancer cases. About 30 percent of cervical cancer cases are caused by other strains of HPV not covered by this vaccine. The two extra strains of HPV in the Gardasil brand account for only about 90 percent of genital warts. About 10 percent of warts are caused by strains not covered by this vaccine. So these vaccines simply make it less likely that a person will catch HPV disease. They are not a guarantee. Neither vaccine helps treat any active HPV warts or cervical disease.

Vaccine manufacturers are continuing to work on new HPV vaccines to incorporate other strains of the virus. As these develop, I will post updates at www.TheVaccineBook.com.

As of the writing of this book, Cervarix hasn't been approved for use, so I can't provide details. The information I'm giving you is for Gardasil only. When Cervarix or other HPV vaccines are approved, I will post specific information at www.TheVaccineBook.com.

HOW IS THE HPV VACCINE MADE?

The Gardasil brand is a genetically engineered vaccine using advanced genetic techniques, similar to how the hep B vaccine is made. Yeast cells (maintained in a solution of vitamins, amino acids, mineral salts, and carbohydrates) are taught to produce the proteins that are found on the outer capsule of four strains of HPV. The yeast cells are broken up and the HPV protein fragments are collected. The proteins are filtered and chemically purified (details on this step are not listed), then combined with aluminum sulfate, water, saline, and a couple of chemicals (see the ingredients list below).

The actual human papillomavirus is never used to make this vaccine. Yeast cells produce the capsule protein, so there's no way to catch HPV disease from this vaccine.

WHAT INGREDIENTS ARE IN THE FINAL VACCINE SOLUTION?

The Gardasil brand contains:

- Proteins from the capsules of 4 strains of HPV
- Aluminum—225 mcg
- Saline solution
- L-histidine (an amino acid)
- Polysorbate 80—50 mcg
- Sodium borate—35 mcg
- Water

Are any of these ingredients controversial?

- Aluminum. This is the only concern with this vaccine. Since the HPV vaccine is given only to older kids, the small amount of aluminum shouldn't be a problem (compared with the risk of giving too much aluminum to a small baby). See pages 193 to 206 for more on aluminum.
- Polysorbate 80. The small amount of polysorbate 80 shouldn't be a problem. See page 209 for more info.

WHAT ARE THE SIDE EFFECTS OF THE HPV VACCINE?

Fever occurs in about 10 percent of people, and the other standard side effects occur in 2 to 5 percent of people.

Birth defects. During initial safety testing of 20,000 women, 2200 became pregnant (half in the vaccine group and half in the placebo control group). Among the vaccinated women, fifteen babies were born with birth defects. Sixteen babies were born with birth defects in the placebo group. This suggests that getting the vaccine while pregnant does not increase the risk of birth defects.

However, for the women who got pregnant within thirty days of getting a vaccine or placebo shot, there were five birth defects in the vaccine group and no birth defects in the placebo group. These defects involved the intestines, kidneys, hips, or feet. This suggests that becoming pregnant within one month of getting the vaccine may increase the risk of birth defects. Extra precautions should be taken to avoid pregnancy during this time period. Further research is being done to evaluate this risk.

Autoimmune side effects. In the 12,000 women who got the vaccine, 9 experienced arthritis side effects that, according to the product insert, may indicate an autoimmune disease. In the 10,000 women who got a placebo shot, only 3 reported such symptoms. Further research will probably be done to evaluate this issue, but this does suggest a very slight risk of autoimmune disease.

I will post updates on www.TheVaccineBook.com when more research becomes available on these side effects.

SHOULD YOU GIVE YOUR CHILD THE HPV VACCINE?

Reasons to get this vaccine

Obviously, a vaccine that decreases the risk of cervical cancer is a wonderful idea, and most parents will probably want this shot for their preteen girls. Genital wart prevention is an added benefit.

People would like to think their daughters won't become sexually active until their honeymoon, but the reality is that some young women and men have sex at a younger age than their parents would hope. Since this usually happens without the parents' knowledge, getting vaccinated well before the possibility exists is a safe precaution.

Since there may be a risk of birth defects if a woman becomes pregnant during the month following the shot, it makes sense to get vaccinated before sexual activity even begins.

Even for women who abstain, the vaccine has benefits. Their new husbands may carry the virus if they didn't choose abstinence before marriage, and the vaccine will help protect these women from contracting HPV disease.

Reasons some people choose not to get this vaccine

Some parents may be cautious, since this is a new vaccine. They may wait a few years to make sure it is safe.

Some parents believe their daughters won't become sexually active until the later teen years or college age. They may therefore choose to delay this shot until that time approaches. A girl who plans to begin having sex in college can get the shot at the college health center without having to tell her parents about it.

Another reason parents might delay the shot is that we are not yet sure how long it lasts. Vaccination at age twelve may not provide protection from HPV all the way through college. We know now that it lasts for at least four years.

A woman who chooses to abstain from sex until marriage does not need this vaccine if the man she marries also chooses abstinence.

This vaccine prevents only the most common strains of HPV. It doesn't protect against other STDs, such as HIV, syphilis, and gonorrhea. Some vaccine critics worry that women who are vaccinated for HPV and hepatitis B may develop a false sense of security and be more likely to have unprotected sex. This puts them at risk for STDs that we don't yet have a vaccine for, including HPV disease strains not covered by this vaccine.

Although this vaccine may reduce or eliminate the most common strains of HPV, some experts worry this might cause the less common strains to become more prevalent.

Travel considerations

There are no travel issues related to this vaccine. A person is just as likely to contract HPV here in the United States as in any other country. Twenty years from now, when, I hope, HPV is reduced or eliminated here, this might be another story.

Options to consider when getting this vaccine

Since the Gardasil brand protects against more strains of HPV than Cervarix, it makes sense to get Gardasil instead. (I bet the Cervarix makers are thinking, "Dang, we should have thought of that!") When the Cervarix data become available, I will post information about the ingredients and side effects on www.TheVaccineBook.com so you and your doctor can compare the two brands.

THE VACCINE BOOK / 152

THE WAY I SEE IT

This vaccine is a fairly good idea. It has the potential to dramatically decrease cervical cancer in our population if it works as well in the general public as it has in the initial trials. Since it is new, however, we don't have a lot of safety data yet. If the safety profile pans out, this will become a very important vaccine. If all preteen girls are vaccinated, eventually these common strains of HPV will stop circulating in our population and the rates of genital warts and cervical cancer should decrease. Unfortunately, there are other strains of HPV out there, and these may increase over the years. Future vaccines will probably incorporate these other strains.

13

Combination Vaccines, Vaccines for Travel, and Vaccines for Other Special Situations

COMBINATION VACCINES

There are twelve separate vaccines on the AAP's recommended schedule, and sometimes as many as six are given at one doctor visit. This can be pretty rough on a little two-month-old baby. You can decrease the number of injections your baby gets by using combination vaccines. Manufacturers have put together several vaccines that combine two or three shots into one. Here are the available combinations to date:

- Chickenpox and MMR—combined as ProQuad (Merck). See page 93.
- DTaP, hep B, and polio—combined as Pediarix (GlaxoSmith-Kline). See page 40.
- DTaP, HIB, and polio—combined as Pentacel (Sanofi Pasteur). See page 40.
- HIB and hep B—combined as Comvax (Merck). See page 11.
- DTaP and HIB—combined as TriHIBit (Sanofi Pasteur). This can be combined for the eighteen-month dose only. It isn't combined for the first three doses. See page 12.

- Hep A and hep B—combined as Twinrix (GlaxoSmithKline). This is for adults eighteen and older only. See page 117.

The manufacturing process and ingredients of most of these shots are identical to the sum of their parts, meaning you get the same dose of the various chemicals and additives as when you get the shots separately. There is one exception to this: Comvax (hep B and HIB mixed) by Merck has only 225 micrograms of aluminum. Given separately, hep B and HIB (using the Merck brands) give your baby 475 micrograms of aluminum.

Many doctors incorporate combo vaccines into their schedule to decrease the number of injections. However, a major drawback to this practice is the total amount of aluminum injected at each visit. When the Pediarix combo is used (DTaP, hep B, and polio), along with separate HIB, Pc, and rota vaccines at the two-, four-, and six-month checkups, the total amount of aluminum at each visit is between 975 and 1200 micrograms. As you will learn in chapter 16, this amount of aluminum greatly exceeds the FDA's safety limit. Some doctors use the Pentacel combo (DTaP, HIB, and polio), along with separate Pc, hep B, and rota vaccines at two, four, and six months. While this mix adds up to only 705 micrograms of aluminum each time, it still exceeds the FDA's safety limit. Even the smaller combo of HIB and hep B in Comvax gives a baby some unnecessary aluminum that could otherwise be avoided by giving an aluminum-free HIB shot and delaying the hep B vaccine for a few years. And ProQuad (MMR and chickenpox) gives a baby four live-virus vaccines at once. I prefer to give only one live-virus vaccine at a time to minimize side effects.

I am not a big fan of combo shots. They don't fit well into my Alternative Vaccine Schedule that you will learn about in chapter 19. I prefer to spread the vaccines out and give less at each visit in order to avoid overloading a baby with so many shots and chemicals at once. I also prefer to use aluminum-free brands whenever possible and only give one aluminum-containing vaccine at a time. When this is done, the amount of aluminum given at any one time can be as low as 125 to 170 micrograms.

If you want to be extra cautious and do only one or two vaccines at a time, most combo vaccines won't be for you. Of course, most parents don't even make these choices. The doctor usually decides which brands to use and what fits in best with the vaccine schedule for the office. I recommend you ask your doctor what, if any, combo vaccines are used. Your doctor may be open to other options if you have a preference. It is fine to switch to any individual vaccines after your baby has already begun a vaccine series with any combo vaccine.

VACCINES FOR TRAVEL

Vaccine recommendations for travel vary each year. You can get the most up-to-date information from www.cdc.gov/travel about which shots you may need to consider when traveling the world. Here is a brief explanation of the three main vaccines that are used for international travel.

Yellow fever vaccine

Yellow fever is a viral disease contracted through mosquitoes, and it is usually fatal. Fortunately it is rare. It occurs mainly in sub-Saharan Africa and the tropical portions of South America (Bolivia, Brazil, Colombia, Ecuador, French Guiana, Guyana, Panama, Paraguay, Peru, Suriname, Trinidad and Tobago, and Venezuela). The vaccine is approved for children nine months of age and older. It is made by growing the yellow fever virus in chicken embryos. The viruses are removed and put into a solution of saline, gelatin, and sorbitol. This vaccine has some very serious side effects, including viscerotropic disease (multiple-organ system failure) and encephalitis (brain inflammation and infection). This occurs because the vaccine contains live viruses, so it can cause an actual infection. These potentially serious side effects are not rare, but since the disease is usually fatal, the shot is still recommended for those traveling to areas where yellow fever is prevalent and mosquito precautions aren't possible.

Typhoid fever vaccine

Typhoid fever is a bacterial salmonella-type illness that is contracted through contaminated water and food in developing countries in Asia, Africa, and Central and South America. Some cases cause only mild intestinal symptoms, but occasionally a person becomes very ill with severe abdominal pain, flu symptoms, and neurologic problems. The disease is treatable with antibiotics.

There are two vaccines indicated for children age two years and older: an oral live-bacterial vaccine and a more commonly used injectable vaccine. The oral form is made by growing the bacteria in non-animal cultures, then placing the whole live bacteria in a capsule with some amino acids and sugars. Four doses are taken over a one-week period. Protection lasts about five years, and the doses can be repeated every five years if travel situations continue. Flu-like side effects can occur, but these are less common than with the injectable form.

The injectable vaccine contains only the sugars that coat the outer shell of the bacteria, phenol, phosphates, and polydimethylsiloxane (try saying that three times fast). Unfortunately, this vaccine doesn't work as well as most routine childhood shots and must be repeated every two years (if repeated travel occurs). About 20 percent of people experience flu-like side effects.

These vaccines are only about 50 to 80 percent effective in preventing typhoid fever, so some people choose not to get this vaccine even when traveling to a risky area.

Japanese encephalitis vaccine

Japanese encephalitis is spread by mosquitoes in Southeast Asia, China, India, and eastern Russia. Most people who catch it don't even notice any symptoms. Those who do become ill, however, suffer severe neurologic problems, and about one in three sufferers will die. Travelers to certain countries who plan to engage in prolonged outdoor activities (such as camping) during seasons of the year when mosquitoes are more prevalent should consider vaccination. This vaccine is made by infecting the brains of mice, then extracting and liquefying the brains. This solution is then sterilized and filtered. The final vaccine solution contains the whole viruses (inactivated with formaldehyde), thimerosal (mercury), formaldehyde, polysorbate 80, and mouse blood proteins. About 10 percent of people suffer fairly unpleasant side effects and about one in two hundred people who get this three-shot series will have a very severe life-threatening allergic reaction.

What about international travelers bringing diseases into the United States? Does this put us at risk? The answer is no. While theoretically a visitor to our country could bring the occasional nasty germ with them, in reality this has rarely happened. This risk isn't significant enough to lose sleep over. What about immigrants? Are those of us living on the border of Mexico more likely to encounter diseases that are virtually eradicated from the United States? Living in Southern California, I get these questions a lot. Again I must answer no. The risk to those of us living in border states is negligible.

VACCINES FOR OTHER SPECIAL SITUATIONS

Rabies vaccine

The rabies virus is contracted through the bite of an animal infected with rabies (usually bats, raccoons, coyotes, and skunks). If the virus is left untreated, rabies is usually fatal once symptoms develop (anxiety, seizures, and paralysis). This usually occurs about two months after a bite, although it can be as soon as five days and as late as one year. The rabies vaccine is given as five injected doses over the month following a high-risk bite. There are two main brands of rabies vaccines used in the United States. In the first one (Imovax by Sanofi Pasteur), the virus is grown and multiplied in a human cell culture. Batches are removed, filtered, and chemically purified. The vaccine solution contains the killed virus, albumin (blood proteins), neomycin (an antibiotic), and phenol. The second brand (RabAvert by Chiron) is made by growing the virus in chicken embryo cells with various chemicals and cow serum (the liquid part of blood). The final filtered product contains the killed virus, polygeline (gelatin made from cow parts), human albumin, glutamate, EDTA, chicken protein, and three antibiotics. Flu-like side effects from the vaccines are common, and some severe neurologic reactions have been reported.

Another type of treatment, called rabies immune globulin, can also be administered if a known exposure to rabies occurs. These rabies antibodies are made by vaccinating healthy volunteers with the rabies vaccine, then taking donated units of their blood and filtering out the rabies antibodies. These antibodies are treated and sterilized with various chemicals and filtering steps. The vaccine solution, containing the antibodies, saline, and glycine (an amino acid), is injected around the wound site to immediately inactivate any rabies virus present. When a person is bitten by an animal known to have rabies, both the vaccine and the immune globulin are given. If the animal is a high-risk rabies animal but not known to actually be rabid, only the vaccine is given while the animal undergoes testing for rabies.

Smallpox vaccine

Routine use of the smallpox vaccine in the United States was stopped in 1969, when the disease was considered eradicated worldwide. Many people born in 1969 or earlier still have a quarter-size scar on the shoulder from this vaccine. After the September 11 terrorist attacks, in 2001, numerous health care workers, emergency workers, and military personnel were given this vaccine so they would be protected in the event of a bioterrorist attack. This practice was halted due to some serious cardiac side effects. At this time, smallpox vaccine will be given only if an attack or outbreak of smallpox occurs. Given the unlikelihood of this event, I have not included specific information in this book.

Anthrax vaccine

An anthrax vaccine is available in the United States, but it is not used for the general public. In the event of a bioterrorist attack, this might be used to contain outbreaks. Since it is not routinely used, I won't include details here.

Tuberculosis skin tests

Every child gets a TB skin test several times throughout childhood. Some doctors begin this at age one, and others wait until a child enters kindergarten. This isn't actually a vaccine at all. Vaccines give a person immunity from a disease. A TB test simply tests to see if a person was ever exposed to tuberculosis and has the TB germs living quietly within the body. Even though this isn't a vaccine, because it uses a needle, some parents and most kids still consider it a "shot."

The TB test solution consists of proteins removed from the tuberculosis germ. These proteins are then put into a solution of saline, polysorbate 80 (only 0.0005 percent of the solution; see page 209 for a discussion of this chemical), and phenol as a preservative.

The solution (0.1 ml) is injected just beneath the skin to form a small bump. The bump quickly fades. If a bump (looking like a mosquito bite) returns within forty-eight to seventy-two hours, this means the person may have a dormant tuberculosis infection that requires evaluation by a doctor. The only side effect reported from TB skin testing is a hypersensitivity reaction at the test site, causing a painful blister.

Tetanus vaccine

Even though I've discussed the tetanus vaccine in detail already, I'm including it here as a reminder for people who get injured. All vaccinated children get enough tetanus shots to cover them in the event of a severe wound for the first twelve to fifteen years of life. Between age twelve and fifteen, a tetanus or the combined Tdap booster is due, which provides another ten years of coverage. A Tdap or plain tetanus booster is recommended every ten years after that, but most adults (meaning myself included) don't remember to keep up with any booster shots. We're just too chicken. I remember getting my last shots in medical school and, I kid you not, two nurses had to chase me around the room (actually, it was kind of fun).

If any child or adult gets a wound that is large, deep, and dirty enough to warrant a trip to an ER, the doctor will want to make certain they are protected from tetanus. Even though booster shots last about ten years, the immunity can wane after five years. So, if it has been more than five years since your last tetanus shot, be prepared to get stuck. And if you've ever wanted to be chased down by a nurse or two, here's your chance.

14

Vaccine Safety Research

Perhaps the most pressing question on every parent's mind is whether vaccines are safe. Most people acknowledge that vaccines are important for preventing disease, and most parents therefore want their kids vaccinated, but they want to know the risks.

No vaccine is completely, 100 percent safe. Each one has potential side effects, some possibly fatal. No one has ever said otherwise. But here's the good news: These severe side effects seem to be extremely rare. Most infants and children go through the standard series of vaccines with few or no apparent problems at all. Yet some vaccine critics believe that there may be side effects that don't show up for years and that the current system for monitoring and discovering such effects is inadequate. Truthfully, when I reviewed all the safety research on vaccines, I found one thing lacking. No one has ever published a thorough statistical analysis on the actual risks of a severe vaccine reaction. We know these reactions happen. We hope they are rare. But what do we actually know for sure? Many studies report on severe reactions, but these data aren't collected into one cohesive package. We don't know the exact number of severe reactions for each vaccine or the frequency of these reactions. Parents need this information. As a doctor, I would love to have it too.

Overall, most studies assert that the benefits of vaccines far outweigh any negative effects. In this chapter, I will give you an in-depth look at the research and provide you with my own statistical analysis. My goal is to help you gain enough understanding to draw your own conclusions about vaccine risk versus benefit.

Vaccines go through two phases of safety testing. In the first phase, thousands of infants and children are given a vaccine in a controlled study (depending on the vaccine, as little as a couple of thousand to as many as thirty thousand). Over several weeks, they are monitored for side effects, which are reported to the FDA. As long as nothing severe commonly shows up, the vaccine is considered safe to use in the general population.

The second phase of safety research is called "postmarketing surveillance." As a vaccine is used in hundreds of thousands of kids in the general population, more side effects begin to arise, some mild and some severe. These effects are reported to the Centers for Disease Control's Vaccine Adverse Events Reporting System (VAERS). When deemed appropriate, these effects are added to the vaccine's product insert. If a vaccine is found to have too high a rate of severe side effects, it is taken off the market, which has happened three times in the past twenty years. The first was the DTP vaccine (an older version of DTaP), which was suspected to cause shock/collapse or extreme high-pitched screaming and high fevers for days. We stopped using it in the late nineties. Next was the live-virus oral polio vaccine, which could actually cause paralysis. We stopped using this vaccine in around the year 2000. The third was the rotavirus vaccine RotaShield. In 1999 research suggested that it might cause life-threatening intestinal blockage after it was given to hundreds of thousands of infants during its first year on the market (newer rotavirus vaccines haven't been proven to cause this dangerous side effect).

Parents considering vaccination want to know what chance their baby has of developing a severe side effect. For the mild, standard side effects like fever and fussiness, the answer is easy, as these effects are carefully calculated during the first phase of safety research (overall, the chance is about 5 to 10 percent with most vaccines, and as high as 40 percent with some). I have detailed this risk in each vaccine chapter.

Unfortunately, when it comes to severe, life-threatening side effects, the actual statistical chances are less clear. The VAERS data tally the reported severe side effects, but nobody has published an accounting of how often these effects occur within a given number of doses of each vaccine. For example, the VAERS database contains information on how many times Guillain-Barré syndrome has occurred after vaccines (see page 181), but we don't know the percentage per doses given. So we can't tell parents, "Your baby has a 0.01 percent chance of having a severe reaction." All we can say is, "Your baby may have a severe reaction, but it is extremely unlikely."

UNDERSTANDING THE STATISTICAL RISK OF A SEVERE VACCINE REACTION

Vaccine critics propose that the risk of a severe vaccine reaction may equal or exceed the risk of having a severe case of a disease. At best, this fear is simply theoretical. I have never found a complete analysis of this issue, one that compares all vaccine-preventable diseases with all severe vaccine reactions. However, I do think that there are enough data available to provide a basic understanding of the likelihood that your child may suffer a severe vaccine reaction. I will also review for you the statistical possibility that your child may suffer a severe case of a vaccine-preventable disease.

A few years ago, the American Academy of Pediatrics newspaper gave an update on vaccine safety based on VAERS data collected by the CDC from 1991 through 2001. It found the following during this ten-year period:

- 1.9 billion doses of vaccines were given in the United States.
- 18,000 severe side effects were reported.
- These effects resulted in a prolonged hospital stay, a severe life-threatening illness, a permanent disability, or death.

These data mean that for about every 100,000 doses, one person suffered a severe reaction (1,900,000,000 divided by 18,000). So the easiest and most straightforward way to answer the question "How likely is it that a baby or child may have a bad reaction to a vaccine?" is about a 1 in 100,000 chance for each dose the child gets.

Let's take these numbers a step further and try to determine a child's risk of a vaccine reaction, not just per dose, but for the entire series of shots throughout childhood.

During the 1990s, when these data were collected, kids got about 18 shots during their childhood (Pc, rotavirus, chickenpox, hepatitis A, meningococcal, HPV, and flu shots weren't routine yet). If you divide 100,000 (the chance of a severe reaction) by 18 (the total number of shots given), there was about a 1 in 5500 chance that any one child might suffer a bad reaction during the entire vaccine schedule in the 1990s.

Let's apply this likelihood of a severe reaction to the number of vaccines given today. If a child gets the 39 total doses of vaccines on the current twelve-year schedule (6 DTaP, 4 HIB, 4 Pc, 3 hep B, 4 polio, 3 rotavirus, 2 MMR, 2 chickenpox, 2 hep A, 1 meningococcal, 3 HPV, and about 5 flu shots), there is a 1 in

2500 chance he will have a severe reaction over the entire twelve-year period (100,000 divided by 39). You can also look at this calculation in a different way. Each time your child gets a shot, there is the 1 in 100,000 chance of a severe reaction. This chance is the same for every shot he gets. Over the twelve-year period, he will be taking this risk 39 times. This analysis is the best I could come up with to determine the likelihood that any one child, or shall we say *your* child, will have a severe, life-threatening reaction.

There is, unfortunately, another way to look at these numbers. I say "unfortunately" because the more ways you try to look at something, the more confusing it can get. I think this approach is valuable, however. I told you that there were 18,000 reactions from 1.9 billion shots. But kids get an average of about 3 shots at a time (39 doses spread out over about 13 doctor visits), so you could argue that these reactions didn't occur from a total of 1.9 billion events (vaccines), but rather from 633 million events or *rounds* of shots (1.9 billion divided by 3). If you divide 633 million events (rounds of vaccines) by 18,000 reactions, you get about a 1 in 35,000 chance of a serious reaction for each *round* of shots—a higher likelihood than the 1 in 100,000 calculated for each individual shot. Doing the math this way suggests that a child takes a 1 in 35,000 risk each time he gets a round of shots, and he takes this risk 13 times. Then divide 35,000 by 13 (the chance of a reaction over all 13 rounds), and you get about a 1 in 2700 chance of a severe reaction throughout childhood. Whew, did I just lose you? Read it again. And again. I had to go through it several times to get it straight.

Looking at the numbers this way, the risk with each round of shots increases. Instead of a 1 in 100,000 chance of a reaction *per vaccine,* it's a 1 in 35,000 chance of a reaction *per round of vaccines.* But each child is taking this risk only 13 instead of 39 times. So in the end, the risk throughout childhood is pretty similar—a 1 in 2500 chance or 1 in 2700 chance, for an average of 1 in 2600.

So let's summarize all that painful math. The risk of a serious vaccine reaction can be calculated as:

- 1 in 100,000 chance for each separate vaccine
- 1 in 35,000 chance for each *round* of vaccines
- 1 in 2600 chance for the entire twelve-year vaccine schedule

Keep in mind that these data are based on only the known reactions that occur close enough to a vaccine for a report to be made. We know that not all vaccine reactions are reported, but we don't know exactly how many go unreported. Is the real number of reactions double what I've put here? Is it triple or more? If so, that would make the chance of a reaction occuring over the entire schedule about 1 in 1300 to 1 in 900. But we don't actually know those numbers, so instead I must work with the numbers that we do know.

The data also don't take into account unknown factors, such as whether vaccines cause chronic, underlying problems. Some vaccine critics worry that conditions like attention–deficit/hyperactivity disorder, autism, learning disorders, neurologic problems, and autoimmune diseases, issues that seem to plague our nation's children much more now than they did twenty years ago, may be triggered in part by the increased number of vaccines given today. If such problems indeed *are* caused by vaccines, then the risk of vaccines would far exceed the risks of the diseases themselves. But there's really no way to determine this risk accurately, because we just don't know if vaccines play a role in these conditions.

One weakness in this analysis is that it is based on data from 1991 through 2001. Now we give babies about twice the number of injections as we did back then. We have some new vaccines, and some older ones have been taken off the market. In order to understand vaccine risks for our kids today, we would need to look at these data using today's vaccine schedule. So far, they aren't available. I hope that in the next revision of this book I will be able to present data from 2001 to 2011 and to do the math for you again.

Besides understanding the overall risk for the complete array of vaccines, many parents naturally want to know the risk for each individual vaccine. Do some vaccines cause severe side effects more often than others? Probably. Does this information exist somewhere? It's in the VAERS database. But VAERS is simply a list of all reported reactions to vaccines. One would have to go through each of the multiple tens of thousands of reactions and separate them by vaccine. And many reactions occur after several simultaneous vaccines. How would we know which vaccine is responsible for the reaction? Someone could probably figure this all out if he had a few years of free time. But I am not that someone. Not with a family and a very busy medical practice. This lack of accessible information is one of the biggest frustrations for parents who are trying to make a decision about vaccines. If you knew which vaccines had the greatest chance of a severe reaction, you might avoid them. If you knew that some vaccines virtually never caused a bad reaction, you would feel very confident in their safety and importance. I truly wish I could make this distinction available to you. All I can offer right now are these overall risks. On pages 186 to 187, I do provide a little bit of insight into determining which vaccines *may* be more reactive than others.

THE STATISTICAL RISK OF SUFFERING A SEVERE CASE OF A VACCINE-PREVENTABLE DISEASE

Now that I've told you the possible risks of a vaccine reaction, what about the statistical chance that your child might get a se-

vere, life-threatening case of one of these *diseases?* To my knowledge, that information has never been determined accurately
through precise scientific statistical analysis. So once again, I will
simply pull out my calculator and attempt to come up with some
useful numbers.

We have good data on the total number of cases of most diseases, as well as the total number of fatalities. But what we don't
know is how often a severe case results in hospitalization or disability but not death. However, we can make some educated as-
sumptions about most of the diseases based on what we know
about each illness and the percent chance each illness usually
causes problems. This information allows us to compare the risks
of severe vaccine reactions (a prolonged hospital stay, a severe
life-threatening illness, a permanent disability, or death) to the
risks of having a severe or fatal case of a disease that could have
been prevented *by* the vaccines. If the chance of being harmed by
one of these diseases was much higher than the chance of a severe
reaction to the shots, then parents would feel more reassured
about the small chance of a vaccine side effect. If, on the other
hand, the chance of severe harm from a disease was much lower
than 1 in 2600 (or 1 in 100,000, or 1 in 35,000, depending on how
you look at it), then parents would be more concerned about the
vaccine itself.

Let's look at the approximate numbers of yearly cases of each
disease in the United States that could be categorized as serious
cases in children twelve and under. I have chosen to examine
these diseases in children instead of in our entire population because it is during childhood that the vaccines are given, and you
are trying to make vaccine decisions for your children, not for
yourself and your parents. (At the end of this section, I will include an analysis that includes both kids and adults.)

Here are the approximate numbers of severe cases of vaccine-
preventable diseases that occur each year in children twelve and

under. In order to be classified as serious, a disease has to require hospitalization, cause permanent disability, or be fatal. I don't consider simple ER visits serious, because ER visits for vaccine reactions aren't part of the tabulated serious reactions. Most of these numbers are fairly accurate based on what we know about each illness and data collected by the *MMWR* (the official CDC disease-reporting system). In some cases, where accurate data don't exist, I've had to make an educated guess. I have made a note next to each number that I've approximated:

- HIB—25 hospitalizations
- Pc—10,000 hospitalizations (very approximate)
- Diphtheria—5 hospitalizations (yearly maximum; some years there are 0)
- Tetanus—5 hospitalizations
- Pertussis—1500 hospitalizations (very approximate)
- Hepatitis B—130 cases, all severe
- Rotavirus—50,000 hospitalizations (approximate)
- Polio—0
- Measles—close to 0
- Mumps—10 hospitalizations (approximate)
- Rubella—3 babies born with defects
- Chickenpox—200 hospitalizations (approximate)
- Hepatitis A—20 hospitalizations (approximate)
- Flu—20,000 hospitalizations (approximate)
- Meningococcal disease—2750 hospitalizations
- HPV—close to 0 until sexual activity begins

This list gives us a very rough total of about 85,000 severe disease cases each year in children. We know that the current U.S. population of kids twelve and under is about 50 million. Dividing 50 million by 85,000 cases means that each child has a 1 in 600 chance of suffering a severe case of a vaccine-preventable illness over the first twelve years of life.

But this isn't a very accurate way to look at disease risk for children. The various diseases affect children in so many different ways at different ages. Some infant diseases occur mainly during the first two years of life and are virtually unheard of beyond that. Some diseases are serious only during the first year of life but are fairly mild when they occur during childhood. Other diseases are mild during young childhood but more severe later on. So it isn't very useful to think of all these diseases in our entire childhood population as a whole.

The most accurate way to assess the risk of having a severe case of a disease is to follow one group of infants throughout their entire childhood and to discuss each disease as it tends to occur at the various ages. I will make this group of kids number 5 million, the number of babies born each year in the United States. Let's put *your* child in this group so you can understand disease risk for him alone. I will now run the numbers on a year's worth of infants from birth through age twelve. For a couple of diseases, I will extend the risk assessment through age twenty-five, because the vaccines given at age twelve are designed to protect against those diseases into young adulthood. I hope to give you a good understanding of disease risk versus vaccine risk for your child. As I explained previously, I don't have precise data on some diseases, so I've had to make some educated guesses.

For clarification, a risk of 1 in 100 means that out of every one hundred people, one person is expected to suffer that event (whether it's a disease or a vaccine reaction). This ratio represents a very high risk. Compare it to a very low risk of only 1 in 100,000, in which it would take a large group of 100,000 people to find one person that would suffer an event.

HIB (meningitis, bloodstream infection). There are about 25 severe cases each year, but most cases occur during the first two years of life. HIB is virtually unheard of beyond that. So during the first two years of these 5 million babies' lives, the risk of a severe case of HIB is about 1 in 200,000 (5 million divided by 25 cases). Beyond age two, the risk is close to 0.

Pc (meningitis, bloodstream infection). There are about 10,000 severe cases each year (this estimate is very rough because the disease is not well reported). It is similar to HIB in that it mainly occurs in the first two years. The disease risk would therefore be about 1 in 500 (5 million divided by 10,000).

Pertussis (whooping cough). With about 1500 severe cases each year in infants (virtually all fatalities and hospitalizations occur in the first six months of life), the severe disease risk would be about 1 in 3333. This risk really applies only to the first year of life.

Rotavirus (diarrhea/dehydration). Very rough estimates put the number of rotavirus hospitalizations at about 50,000 per year. This number gives our babies about a 1 in 100 risk of a severe case. Rotavirus is rarely severe beyond age two.

Flu (. . . flu . . .). There are about 20,000 severe cases each year in infants (a fairly rough estimate). This number puts the severe disease risk at about 1 in 250 during the first two years, when the flu is most risky for kids. For older kids and young adults, flu hospitalizations are very rare. With only about 50 fatalities reported each year (see page 122), I would estimate 2000 hospitalizations. This calculation gives us a disease risk of about 1 in 2500 for children and young adults.

Meningococcal disease (meningitis). About 2500 cases occur in our infants during the first two years of life, putting the disease risk at about 1 in 2000 during infancy. Another 250 cases occur between then and the preteen years, giving our kids a disease risk of 1 in 20,000. The vaccine isn't yet available for kids during childhood, so this risk is unavoidable for now. In the near future, we may start using this vaccine for two-year-olds. Only about another 250 cases occur each year during the teen and college years. So from age twelve, when the vaccine is currently given, the disease risk is only about 1 in 20,000.

Let me point out that these first six diseases are responsible for the vast majority of serious infant disease cases. The disease risks are mainly worrisome for the first two years or so. For the rest of childhood and into the adult years, these diseases have a much lower risk of being serious.

Now let's move on to the remaining ten diseases, which apply more to later childhood and adulthood:

Hepatitis B (liver disease). According to the actual number of reported cases, we may expect about 130 cases of this disease in our group of 5 million kids over the first twelve years of life. That's a disease risk of about 1 in 40,000. Among teens and college-age kids, when contracting hep B becomes a greater possibility, about 1300 cases are reported each year. This number puts the disease risk at about 1 in 4000. As stated on page 50, however, the true risk may be much higher.

Chickenpox. About 200 serious cases may be expected to occur in our group over the first twelve years. The severe disease risk would be about 1 in 25,000. For teens and young adults, for whom chickenpox is more serious, we may see another estimated 200 serious cases yearly, with a similar risk.

Tetanus. This disease is virtually unheard of in the first five years of life. We see only about 10 cases annually among those who are between ages five and twenty-five, giving us a disease risk of only about 1 in 500,000.

Diphtheria. This illness is so rare that I put the risk at close to 0 for all age groups.

Measles, mumps, and rubella. Severe cases during childhood are so rare that this risk is close to 0. Just for argument's sake, however, we can use the 20 hospitalizations during the 2006 mumps epidemic to give us a mumps disease risk of 1 in 250,000 for teens and young adults. We can also use the 3 known cases of babies born with rubella birth defects each year to establish a severe disease risk of about 1 in 1.6 million.

Hepatitis A (temporary liver disease). Severe cases in children are extremely rare. In teens and young adults, we may see about 200 severe cases yearly, putting the risk for the older group at about 1 in 25,000.

Polio. This disease doesn't occur in our country, so the risk is 0 for all age groups.

HPV (genital warts). This virus doesn't occur in children, so the risk is 0 until sexual activity begins. To determine a statistical severe disease risk for teens and young adults, however, is very difficult. Almost every sexually active person contracts this virus at a young age. While most cases won't immediately seem serious, the lifelong implications of carrying HPV in the cervix could be viewed as serious for every woman. The number of teens and young adults who contract problematic genital warts from HPV each year is unknown, but can be estimated. Cervical cancer typically doesn't happen until later in life, but if we consider the number of adult women who eventually have a serious case of

HPV warts or cervical cancer, we can estimate about 20,000 cases each year. This calculation gives a disease risk of about 1 in 250.

As you can see, the risks vary greatly when we compare serious infant diseases with the rest of the childhood ones. In most cases, the childhood and young adult disease risks are much lower than the disease risks during infancy. Does this mean that the vaccines for older children are less important? Not necessarily. Vaccinating keeps these diseases at low levels in our population so we remain at low risk. If older kids are vaccinated, it lowers the risk that they'll pass on these diseases to infants. Vaccination also provides some immunity through the teen years and into young adulthood, when some of these diseases *do* become more of a risk.

Now, as we watch our 5 million kids grow up, how do we weigh the severe disease risk against the risk that they will suffer a severe reaction to a vaccine? I told you previously that I don't know how many severe reactions have occured with each of these vaccines individually. I share your frustration that the VAERS database may have the information we need to understand the exact risk of reactions to individual vaccines but that these data aren't accessible. We know that some vaccines cause more severe reactions than others. Some have severe reaction rates that are much higher than 1 in 100,000, while others are lower. An older vaccine was taken off the market in the late 1990s (DTP; see page 35) because the risk of a severe reaction (seizures or sudden shock) was a frightening 1 in 1600 doses. It doesn't seem that any of today's vaccines have a risk even close to this ratio. I hope someday to make detailed information available to you. For now, all I can offer is the overall risk of a vaccine reaction.

For those of you who just can't get enough math and statistics, here's one last page of excitement. What follows is a risk estimate for the incidence of severe cases of a disease over a lifetime in our population as a whole:

- HIB—25 hospitalizations
- Pc—30,000 hospitalizations
- Diphtheria—5 hospitalizations (yearly maximum; some years there are 0)
- Tetanus—100 hospitalizations
- Pertussis—1500 hospitalizations (very approximate)
- Hepatitis B—7500 cases
- Rotavirus—50,000 hospitalizations (approximate)
- Polio—0
- Measles—close to 0
- Mumps—20 hospitalizations (during a recent outbreak)
- Rubella—3 babies born with defects
- Chickenpox—1000 hospitalizations (approximate)
- Hepatitis A—200 hospitalizations (approximate)
- Flu—100,000 hospitalizations (approximate)
- Meningococcal disease—3000 cases
- HPV—20,000 new cases of cervical cancer each year and (very approximate) number of problematic genital wart cases each year

Adding up these numbers, we get approximately 200,000 serious cases of vaccine-preventable diseases each year. We have about 300 million people in the United States. So each person in this country has a 1 in 1500 chance of suffering a severe case of a vaccine-preventable disease each year (300 million divided by 200,000).

Okay. You probably have way too many numbers bouncing around in your head right now, so I'll summarize the highlights of this discussion:

- The risk of a reaction from a single vaccine seems to be about 1 in 100,000.

- The risk that any one child will suffer a severe reaction over the entire twelve-year vaccine schedule is about 1 in 2600.

- The risk of any one person suffering a severe case of a vaccine-preventable disease each year in our entire population is about 1 in 1500.

- The risk of a child having a severe case of a vaccine-preventable disease is about 1 in 600 each year for all childhood diseases grouped together. This risk varies widely depending on the disease. Some disease risks are close to 0. Infant diseases are more risky than childhood ones.

- We don't know the exact number of serious vaccine reactions, as many are likely to go unreported or are not recognized. We also don't know how to factor in possible long-term, hidden effects of vaccines. If we someday can learn these numbers, the known vaccine risk may increase.

So we come back to our original question: Are vaccines safe? Yes. Do they have severe side effects? Yes. Are these severe side effects common? Not very. Is vaccinating to protect against all these diseases worth the risk of side effects? That's the million-dollar question. I have given you the best possible analysis based on the data that are available to me at this time so that you can make your own informed decision.

INADEQUATE LONG-TERM SAFETY RESEARCH?

Besides trying to assess vaccine versus disease risk, critics of vaccines cite another major issue when it comes to safety research. They worry that each new vaccine that comes out isn't adequately researched for long-term safety. For example, a new medication goes through many years of trials in a select group of people to make sure it is safe. These subjects undergo extensive blood testing and physical evaluations over many years. If nothing severe or common shows up, the medication is then released for general use.

Vaccines, on the other hand, don't receive the same type of in-depth short-term testing or long-term safety research. The original test subjects aren't monitored for many years to see if any long-term side effects develop. Their blood isn't tested to check for internal toxic effects. Doctors don't do physical exams to look for problems. Most vaccine side effects are monitored via parent questionnaires. Critics worry that many chronic diseases and other physical and mental problems like ADHD, chronic fatigue, diabetes, allergies, asthma, learning disorders, and autism are triggered by vaccines. I haven't found any solid research to support this contention. When I reviewed numerous studies, I did find some that show a possible link between a vaccine and a chronic disease. Examples include the HIB vaccine and diabetes, the hep B vaccine and multiple sclerosis and rheumatoid arthritis, and the MMR vaccine and eczema and chronic arthritis (see "Resources," page 252). However, I also found many studies that conclude that there isn't enough evidence to prove a link, and these studies are definitely in the majority. But there is something missing from all this research. It is limited to animal studies, population comparisons between countries that use a vaccine and those that don't, and analysis of reported reactions (which can't be proven to be caused by a vaccine). No one has simply followed a selected group of vaccine test subjects for twenty years to see what problems develop.

In the heading of this section, I used the term "inadequate." I didn't choose that word at random. I pulled it from a mainstream medical journal, *Vaccine,* which studied the MMR-autism connection. The report concluded that there was no link between the two, but the doctors in the study stated that "the design and reporting of safety outcomes in MMR vaccine studies, both pre- and post-marketing, are largely inadequate." (See "Resources," page 256.)

Vaccine safety researchers face many difficulties. When a new vaccine comes out, they add it to the current series in a test group and compare the side effects with those that the existing vaccines are known to cause. If any new or more common reactions occur, researchers assume that they are from the new vaccine. It's not possible to test a new vaccine by itself, without giving the other routine vaccines at the same time. Virtually every vaccine product insert states that the vaccine was tested alongside existing vaccines, not in isolation.

The only foolproof way to study the long-term side effects of vaccines would be to take 50,000 infants, set aside 10,000 as an unvaccinated control group, and give the remaining four groups of 10,000 babies each a series of only one vaccine. Then testers would follow these kids for twenty years and compare the types of problems they have. Of course, we can never follow this plan, as it would leave many children unvaccinated and susceptible. We could look for 10,000 volunteer families and compare the health of their unvaccinated kids to a group of 10,000 fully vaccinated kids over a twenty-year period. That would be a bit easier. Any volunteers?

Overall, vaccines are generally safe, with some common but mild side effects and some serious but very rare reactions. We know that the diseases themselves can kill. Death and permanent disability from diseases would be a significant problem if we didn't have vaccinations. When vaccines do cause occasional serious permanent reactions, that is tragic. Let's hope that we can make vaccines safer in the future as better techniques develop and more research is done. For now, it's up to you to understand the entire issue as thoroughly as possible so you can feel comfortable with your choices.

15

Vaccine Side Effects

STANDARD SIDE EFFECTS OF VACCINES

Throughout this book I have mentioned some very serious (but very rare) side effects unique to certain vaccines. There are some common reactions, however, that can occur with virtually every vaccine. I call them "standard side effects" because they typically occur about 5 to 10 percent of the time for most shots. Some vaccines cause these reactions as much as 40 percent of the time. Fortunately, these side effects are usually harmless in the long run, and even in the short run. They include, but are not limited to:

- Pain, redness, and swelling at the injection site
- Fever
- Crying
- Vomiting
- Diarrhea
- Poor appetite
- Sleepiness
- Headaches

- Body aches
- Pea-size nodule at injection site lasting for several weeks
- Rash over the whole body or limited to one area

These effects can usually be minimized by holding a cool washcloth or ice pack to the injection site and giving ibuprofen (acetaminophen can also be used, although it may not work as well). See "Is There Any Way to Take the Sting out of Shots?" page 215.

SERIOUS SIDE EFFECTS OF VACCINES

All vaccines have some potentially serious side effects. Fortunately, they are extremely rare. Most of the potential severe reactions that I've listed throughout the book are self-explanatory (or I provided a brief explanation where needed). Here is a discussion of some of the more complicated reactions:

Guillain-Barré syndrome. The body's immune system attacks the nervous system, causing temporary weakness and some paralysis. The effect usually wears off after several weeks, but a person must receive intensive care in the meantime to support the body systems that aren't working (including respiration), and this illness is potentially fatal. It has been reported after various vaccines, although no one has proven that the vaccines actually caused the reaction. The product inserts of some tetanus-containing vaccines (see page 35) state that there is enough evidence to say the vaccines can cause this reaction. This condition also strikes for no apparent reason, even when no vaccines were recently given.

Encephalitis/encephalopathy. Rarely, a baby will register a high fever and scream intensely, alternating with lethargy for several hours and possibly days. This reaction is thought to be due to swelling and inflammation of the brain, the medical term for which is "encephalitis." Virtually all infants with an encephalitis reaction recover without any problems. Unfortunately, a small percentage of cases will progress to *encephalopathy,* during which the brain actually suffers some permanent damage. We don't know for sure if the reaction is caused by vaccination or if it's just coincidental. It seemed to be most commonly associated with the old DTP vaccine, which we no longer use in the United States. The MMR and all tetanus-containing vaccines (according to their product inserts) may also be linked to this reaction.

Subacute sclerosing panencephalitis (SSPE). I already introduced you to this reaction along with the MMR vaccine (page 90). It is similar to encephalitis, but it's more gradual and chronic. Brain function slowly deteriorates over many years. SSPE has various causes, including certain viral infections. We don't know for sure that any vaccine causes it.

Sudden infant death syndrome (SIDS). Do vaccines cause SIDS? This is a lingering question, and the answer is probably no. The main challenge in researching SIDS is that in many cases the baby would have recently received one or more vaccines. The only way to answer this question would be to compare the rate of SIDS in an unvaccinated infant population to the rate in a vaccinated population. But there aren't enough unvaccinated babies for a valid study. Statistical analysis has shown no link between vaccines and SIDS. Some point out that the SIDS rate is lower in a few countries that don't use as many vaccines, but there are so many other differential factors among these countries that the studies aren't really sound. We may never know for sure. See "Resources" to review studies showing a possible link between the old (and no longer used) DTP vaccine and SIDS (page 265) as well as studies showing that DTP does *not* cause SIDS (page 266).

Autism. A possible connection between autism and vaccines is on the mind of every parent today. I have already shared the debate over the MMR vaccine and autism on page 94. But what about the rest of the vaccines? It would take an entire book to discuss this issue thoroughly, but I will try to sum it up in just a few sentences.

Here is what we do know, or suspect, about the causes of autism. Research at Harvard, Johns Hopkins, the University of Arkansas, and the University of California at Davis, to name a few, shows that many autistic kids have a variety of similar health problems, including intestinal disease, autoimmune disease, allergies, brain inflammation, and metabolic defects, as well as a genetic inability to detoxify their bodies of the host of chemicals in food, water, and pollution that are part of our modern society. Their brains and bodies may be affected by the buildup of these environmental chemicals.

The question is: Are the chemicals in vaccines creating enough exposure to contribute to this damage or not? Will we ever answer this hypothesis? Honestly, I don't see how we can. We would need a control group of many thousands of unvaccinated kids to compare with a group of vaccinated kids. Even then, it might be hard to prove a connection. Some studies have been published in recent years that have failed to show statistical proof of a relationship between vaccines and autism. However, by the same token, it is also difficult to prove that there is *not* a connection. As more research becomes available, I will post updates on www.TheVaccineBook.com. But don't expect to find a conclusion to this issue any time soon, if ever.

WHAT TO DO IF YOUR CHILD HAS A VACCINE REACTION

Mild reactions

If your child experiences the standard side effects of fussiness, mild fever, body aches, or mild redness at the injection site, you don't have to do anything but offer a little tender loving care. Such effects will subside over a day or two. Even if your child has a fever over 101, but isn't too fussy or bothered by it, you don't have to offer treatment.

If your child has a fever over 101 and is extremely fussy, I suggest you go ahead and give her some ibuprofen (Motrin or Advil). Acetaminophen (Tylenol) also helps but may not work quite as well for vaccine reactions. Ibuprofen will also address body aches and swelling and redness at the injection site.

Sometimes the arm or leg where the injection is given becomes unusually swollen and/or red. During the first day or two of this reaction, there usually isn't any treatment that your doctor can offer. Simply apply a cold washcloth or ice pack for about ten minutes every hour. You can also give your child ibuprofen to help minimize the redness and swelling, and diphenhydramine (Benadryl, an over-the-counter antihistamine) to help with any allergic reaction. Arnica, a homeopathic remedy for swelling, may also help. It's available at health food stores in oral or topical form. If the redness continues to progress for more than two days, this may mean the injection site has become infected. See a doctor right away.

A rash is not uncommon. It may be a mild allergic reaction during the day or two after the shot or a manifestation of the vaccine germs causing a mild case of the disease itself if it occurs a week or two after injection. In most cases, treatment isn't necessary. Call your doctor if your child seems uncomfortable. If the rash looks like allergic hives (raised white and red welts), give diphenhydramine (Benadryl). Call your doctor if your child's allergic reaction worsens.

Vomiting, diarrhea, poor appetite, and sleepiness are other common reactions, but they don't have any specific treatment.

Severe reactions

If any of the mild reactions don't respond to treatment, or if your child is acting seriously ill, you should call your doctor right away. In most cases, there is no more treatment to offer other than what I've suggested, but it is prudent to have your child evaluated. If you believe your child may be having an encephalitis reaction, using ibuprofen as well as vitamins A and C as suggested on page 189 may help decrease the reaction as you seek medical attention.

REPEATING VACCINES AFTER A SERIOUS REACTION

Surprisingly to me, most vaccine guidelines state that a vaccine series should be continued, even after a serious reaction has occurred, because the benefit of disease protection outweighs the risk of another bad reaction. This thinking may be logical for severe diseases such as meningitis, but does not make sense for very rare or mild diseases. You should carefully review the disease information if your child has a severe reaction and decide along with your doctor if the disease is severe and common enough to warrant repeating the vaccine. Severe reactions tend to become even worse with subsequent shots. So if you do decide to repeat a reactive vaccine, I suggest giving it by itself without any other simultaneous vaccines. The vaccine product inserts do state that a vaccine should not be repeated if a child suffers a severe allergic reaction. Your doctor can give you a medical exemption letter if he or she decides a vaccine shouldn't be repeated.

If your child does have a life-threatening reaction, you should carefully consider whether or not to continue *any* vaccines at all. I know this would leave your child susceptible to many diseases, but the chance of a repeat severe reaction is considerable. I was shocked to read that one of the Guillain-Barré victims of the meningococcal vaccine (not a fatal case, fortunately) had had this reaction in the past with other vaccines. I believe that such a severe reaction should preclude subsequent vaccinations.

RATING THE "REACTIVITY" OF VACCINES

All vaccines are not created equal. Some are more likely to cause reactions. I call these vaccines "reactive" (very insightful of me, huh?). Some vaccines, on the other hand, rarely cause side effects. No one has actually done the scientific research to put all vaccines in exact order of reactivity, but based on my own observations and reading over the years, here is how I would rate vaccines from least reactive to most reactive:

- HIB
- Polio
- DTaP
- Pc
- Chickenpox
- Hepatitis B
- Hepatitis A
- MMR
- Meningococcal
- Flu

The rotavirus and HPV vaccines are too new for me to have formed an impression. I would probably place them somewhere in the middle.

What are the implications of vaccine reactivity? I don't know, and neither does anyone else. Some vaccine opponents worry that vaccines that have a higher rate of fevers, irritability, and other reactions are more likely to cause some sort of permanent injury. This relationship hasn't been shown in any large research studies. However, the whole-cell DTP vaccine was reformulated into the safer DTaP vaccine in the mid-1990s, and the DTP vaccine is no longer used in the United States because of its high level of reactivity, including fever, irritability, lethargy, and seizures. Some kids may have suffered permanent brain injury (see "Resources" for scientific articles that show this may be true, page 265), although this connection hasn't been proven. DTP seems to have been one of the most "reactive" vaccines ever.

NATIONAL VACCINE INJURY COMPENSATION PROGRAM (VICP)

This program is based on a series of laws created in 1986 that allow people who are injured by a vaccine to seek monetary compensation of up to $250,000. The laws also protect the vaccine manufacturers from litigation. It is funded by taxes placed on the purchase of vaccines. The program details are beyond the scope of this book, but you can find them at the U.S. Department of Health and Human Services Web site, www.hrsa.gov/vaccinecompensation.

BOOSTING THE IMMUNE SYSTEM TO PREVENT INFECTIOUS DISEASES AND TO MINIMIZE VACCINE SIDE EFFECTS

A healthy immune system is the key to preventing infectious diseases. We are all exposed to millions of germs every day, and vaccines cover only a tiny fraction of 1 percent of these germs. So we must rely on our own immune system to fight off most potential infections. Children and adults with healthy immune systems are also less likely to suffer a serious vaccine reaction. Most vaccine side effects involve the immune system reacting poorly to the vaccine, so ensuring a healthy immune system is one way parents can decrease their child's risk of a vaccine reaction. Here's what you can do:

Breastfeed. If you are breastfeeding, plan to do so for a minimum of one year. Two years is better. Not only will your baby catch fewer illnesses, but her immune system may be better equipped to handle vaccines. No one has actually studied whether breast-fed babies show fewer reactions, but theoretically it makes sense.

Minimize sugar and junk food. We do know that sugar weakens the immune system—one of the busiest times in our office is the week after Halloween. Of course, this advice doesn't apply to babies, but you should minimize treats and sugary foods for older kids for several weeks prior to checkups and vaccines at the doctor's office.

Minimize other chemical exposures. The small amounts of chemicals in vaccines are unavoidable. But there are other areas of life where we can control this exposure, and one is the foods we feed our kids. Serve organic foods as much as possible, beginning with baby foods. A little baby's growing brain and developing immune system are very susceptible to chemical influences. Eating organic fruits, veggies, grains, and meats is a good way to help ensure a healthier brain and body.

Use omega-3 oil supplements. Most children are deficient in the healthful omega-3 fats, because the main dietary source is fish and eggs, foods that most kids don't eat enough of. Breast milk is also full of omega 3s. Fish oils (in liquid form for toddlers over age one and chewables or capsules for older kids) that are tested and found to be mercury free are a nutritious addition to any diet and can improve many aspects of a child's health, including the immune system.

Probiotics. These healthful bacteria live in our intestines. They play a critical role in regulating both our intestinal immune system and our internal immune system. Antibiotic use, which is a typical part of every infant and child's early life, destroys these bacteria, leaving a child more susceptible to a host of illnesses and intestinal problems. Taking probiotics on a continuous basis, but especially for a week before and several weeks after vaccinations, can really do wonders for the immune system and may help protect from the side effects of vaccines. Also called "acidophilus," probiotics come in liquid or powder form that can be mixed into food or liquid for infants two months and older, or swallowed as small capsules or pearls by older kids.

Fruits and vegetables. Everyone knows these foods are good for you, but unfortunately very few children get enough. Fruit, veggie, and berry supplements are available as chewables for children and as capsules for adults. Infants age one and older can also use the contents of adult capsules mixed into their food. The immune-boosting fruit, veggie, and berry supplements can help prevent infectious diseases and may limit vaccine reactions.

Vitamin A. This specific vitamin helps with neurologic health. It also helps regulate the immune system's response to infections. Some researchers believe it can play a role in protecting the brain from vaccine side effects. Give vitamin A once a day for three days prior to vaccines and continue each day for ten days after. Infants should get 1500 IUs daily, toddlers and preschoolers

2500 IUs, and older kids and teens 5000 IUs. The most commonly available form of vitamin drops for babies and young kids is a mix of vitamins A, C, and D or a multivitamin drop with A, B, C, D, and E. They are available at any drugstore. A better source of vitamin A is cod liver oil, available at health food stores. The label will tell you how much vitamin A is in each teaspoon. You should be aware that overdosing vitamin A can be toxic, so do not exceed the suggested amounts. Don't give cod liver oil to any baby younger than nine months because of the risk of triggering a fish allergy.

Vitamin C. This antioxidant vitamin can help boost the immune system and may decrease vaccine side effects. Give it once a day for five days starting on the day of the shots. Infants should get 150 milligrams daily, toddlers and preschoolers 250 milligrams, and older kids and teens 500 milligrams. Vitamin C drops, chewables, and capsules are available at any health food store or drugstore. The amount of vitamin C in multivitamin drops (combined with vitamin A) usually isn't enough.

Visit www.TheVaccineBook.com for more specific information on boosting your child's immune system and to find out where to buy these types of supplements.

16

Vaccine Ingredients

Everyone has heard that vaccine manufacturers use some unusual components, and some of these ingredients are in the final products. Mercury has probably gotten the most bad press in recent years, and it has finally been removed from most vaccines. But various aspects of vaccine production and ingredients still worry some parents.

ANIMAL AND HUMAN TISSUES

Critics of vaccines point out that some vaccines use human and/or animal tissues in the manufacturing process. I have detailed these for you throughout the book. But are they a big deal? Is there any problem with using these tissues? Well, there *was* a very serious problem that occurred decades ago.

In August 2002 and February 2003 a popular pediatric news publication, *Infectious Diseases in Children,* published reports from experts across the country who met to discuss this issue. Between 1955 and 1963, some of the monkey kidney cells used for the injected polio vaccine, the oral polio vaccine, and the adenovirus vaccine (used for the military; see "Resources," page 268) were contaminated with SV-40 virus, which is known to cause several types of brain tumors, bone cancer, lymphoma, and mesothelioma cancer in animals. This virus has also been discovered in these same cancers in humans. The SV-40 viruses present in some human tumors today have been determined to be genetically identical to those in vaccines fifty years ago. Although the SV-40 virus is found in human tumors, it is not known if the virus causes the tumors or just happens to be living within the tumors. It is known, however, that the virus triggers these tumors in animals. It is estimated that almost 30 million people were injected with a vaccine containing this virus during that eight-year period. Statistical population studies have not shown that these 30 million people had any higher rates of these cancers than the general population. In 1980, 150 newborns were given a hepatitis A vaccine that also was contaminated with the SV-40 virus.

Monkey kidney cells are still used to make the polio vaccine. Numerous other animal and human tissues are used in many vaccines. Now we know to test the monkeys to make sure they are free of SV-40 virus and other known viruses, so the polio vaccine used today is safer. All animal and human tissues are carefully screened for all known infectious diseases. Some vaccine critics are still worried, however, that there may be other viruses or other infectious agents (called "prions," "slow viruses," or "virus particles") that are much smaller than viruses and that we don't yet know how to screen for. Mad cow disease (a rare brain-wasting condition that can affect humans) is one such agent, and we didn't even know it existed until the 1980s. We'd been using cow tissues to make vaccines for decades before that. Were humans injected with that prion? Critics worry that we will discover such contamination in the future, just as the SV-40 virus contamination was found long after the fact. They worry that the human and animal tissues used to make a variety of vaccines may harbor some unknown infectious particles or that the foreign DNA in these tissues may cause problems when injected. At this time, I can't offer any good evidence to support these worries, and I hope I never find any.

For review, here is a list of the various animal or human tissues used to make vaccines:

- Human blood proteins (albumin)
- Human lung cells
- Human fetal lung cells
- Human cell lines
- Cow serum (the liquid part of blood)
- Cow heart-muscle extract
- Cow tissue extract
- Monkey kidney cells
- Guinea pig embryo cells
- Chicken embryos
- Chicken kidney cells
- Chicken eggs

ALUMINUM

Aluminum is added to a number of vaccines to help them work better. Normally one wouldn't consider aluminum to be a problem. It's present everywhere in our environment. It's in food, water, air, and soil. It's also a main ingredient in over-the-counter antacids. Aluminum is thought to be harmless when swallowed because it isn't absorbed into the body.

I didn't think much about aluminum when I first started researching vaccines thirteen years ago. In fact, my early seminars on vaccine education included a brief statement that aluminum was nothing to worry about. So why am I writing about it here?

VACCINES THAT USE ANIMAL OR HUMAN TISSUES

MMR
Chickenpox
Polio
Rotavirus
Flu
Hepatitis A
DTaP (Infanrix and Tripedia brands)
Tetanus and diphtheria vaccines
Tdap (Boostrix brand)

VACCINES THAT *DON'T* USE ANIMAL OR HUMAN TISSUES

HIB
Pc
Hepatitis B
Meningococcal
HPV
DTaP (Daptacel brand)
Tdap (Adacel brand)

As I read each product insert and looked at the micrograms of aluminum in several of the vaccines, I wondered, Has anyone determined a safe level of injected aluminum? I didn't have to wonder for long because I found the answer quite easily. You can find it as well; just go to www.fda.gov and search for "aluminum toxicity." You'll see several documents about aluminum. See also "Resources," pages 250 to 252.

The first document I came across discusses labeling of aluminum content in injected dextrose solutions (a sugar solution added to hospital IVs). On page 2, section 3a, you will read the following:

Aluminum may reach toxic levels with prolonged parenteral administration [injection] if kidney function is impaired. . . . Research indicates that patients with impaired kidney function, including premature neonates, who received parenteral levels of aluminum at greater than 4 to 5 micrograms per kilogram of body weight per day, accumulate aluminum at levels associated with central nervous system and bone toxicity [for a tiny newborn, this toxic dose would be 10 to 20 micrograms, and for an adult it would be about 350 micrograms]. Tissue loading may occur at even lower rates of administration.

Wow, that's a mouthful. I had to read it three times to understand it, so feel free to do the same.

The second document discusses aluminum content in IV feeding solutions (called TPN). The FDA requires these solutions to limit aluminum to 25 micrograms per liter. A typical adult in the hospital would get about 1 liter of TPN solution each day, thus about 25 micrograms of aluminum. The document also states on page 2,

Aluminum content in parenteral drug products could result in a toxic accumulation of aluminum in individuals receiving TPN therapy. Research indicates that neonates and patient populations with impaired kidney function may be at high risk of exposure to unsafe amounts of aluminum. Studies show that aluminum may accumulate in the bone, urine, and plasma of infants receiving TPN. Many drug products used in parenteral therapy [injections] may contain levels of aluminum sufficiently high to cause clinical manifestations [symptoms] . . . parenteral aluminum bypasses the protective mechanism of the GI tract and aluminum circulates and is deposited in human tissues. Aluminum toxicity is difficult to identify in infants because few reliable techniques are available to evaluate bone metabolism in . . . infants. . . . Although aluminum toxicity is not commonly detected clinically, it can be serious in selected patient populations, such as neonates, and may be more common than is recognized.

Okay, that was another mouthful . . . or a syringeful if you prefer. So what does it mean? Here's your translation. According to the first document, if premature babies get more than 10 micrograms of aluminum per day in their IV solution, it may accumulate in their bones and brain at toxic levels. According to the second document, aluminum toxicity is *not* rare in newborns and other patients receiving injectable medications and IV solutions containing aluminum. The report also warns that toxicity is difficult to detect just by observing symptoms.

ASPEN (the American Society for Parenteral and Enteral Nutrition, not the ski resort), a group that monitors for safety and side effects of oral and injectable nutritional products, has also put out a paper on this topic. ASPEN's statement on aluminum safety, published in *Nutrition in Clinical Practice* in 2004 (see "Resources," page 251), reports that aluminum accumulation in body tissues can occur in newborns receiving IV solutions containing aluminum for prolonged periods. It also says that the significance of this fact is not known. The group reiterates the FDA's recommendations that IV nutritional solutions contain no more than 25 micrograms of aluminum per liter. Other injectable products aren't required to limit aluminum, but they are required to have a warning label that says, "This product contains aluminum that may be toxic." The label goes on to specify the worries about aluminum in patients with kidney problems and premature babies and the limit of 5 micrograms per kilogram of body weight per day. ASPEN recommends that doctors "may want to purchase equivalent products with the lowest aluminum content when possible and should monitor changes in the pharmaceutical market that may affect aluminum concentrations."

Where does the 4 to 5 microgram per kilogram per day safety limit come from? I found a very interesting 1997 study in *The New England Journal of Medicine* (see "Resources," page 251) that compared the neurologic development of about one hundred premature babies who were given a standard intravenous feeding solution that contained aluminum with a hundred premature babies who were given the same solution but with almost all the aluminum purposely filtered out. What prompted this study (according to its introduction) was the knowledge that aluminum can build up to toxic levels in the bloodstream, bones, and brain when injected, that preemies have decreased kidney function and have a higher risk of toxicity, that one preemie with sudden, unexplained death had high aluminum concentrations in the brain on autopsy, and that toxicity can cause progressive dementia. So these researchers sought to prove that aluminum may be harmful to preemie babies. They turned out to be right. The infants who were given IV solutions with aluminum showed impaired neurologic and mental development at eighteen months, compared to the babies who were fed much lower amounts of aluminum. Those who got aluminum received an average of about 500 micrograms spread out over an average of 10 days, or about 50 micrograms per day. The babies who got the solution with aluminum filtered out received about 10 micrograms daily, or 4 to 5 micrograms per kilogram of body weight per day.

Now, none of these documents or studies mention vaccines. They look only at IV solutions and injectable medications. I'm not sure why that is. Nor is it clear why the FDA does not require aluminum warning labels on vaccines when it does require a warning on all other injectable medications. Vaccines apparently have some sort of exemption.

All these warnings seem to apply mainly to premature babies

and kidney patients. What about larger, full-term babies with healthy kidneys? Using the 5 microgram per kilogram per day criterion from the first FDA document as a *minimum* amount we know a healthy baby can handle, a twelve-pound, two-month-old baby can safely get at least 30 micrograms of aluminum in one day. A twenty-two-pound one-year-old can get at least 50 micrograms safely. Babies with healthy kidneys could probably handle a lot more, but it's useful to have a benchmark. However, the documents don't tell us what the maximum safe dose would be for a healthy baby or child. And I can't find such information anywhere. This is probably why ASPEN suggests, and the FDA requires, that all injectable solutions have the 25-microgram limit, which we know is safe.

But wait. You are probably thumbing back through the book right now to see exactly how much aluminum was in each vaccine. Put your thumb away. At the risk of being repetitive, I'll list them right here:

- HIB (PedVaxHIB brand only)—225 micrograms per shot
- Pc—125 micrograms
- DTaP—depending on the manufacturer, 170 to 625 micrograms
- Hepatitis B—250 micrograms
- Hepatitis A—250 micrograms
- HPV—225 micrograms
- Pentacel (DTaP, HIB, and polio combo vaccine)—330 micrograms
- Pediarix (DTaP, Hep B, and polio combo vaccine)—850 micrograms

Okay, I'll do the math for you. A newborn who gets a hepatitis B injection on day one of life would get 250 micrograms of aluminum. This dosage would be repeated at one month of age with the next hep B shot. When a baby gets the first big round of shots at two months, the total dose of aluminum can vary from 295 micrograms (if a nonaluminum HIB and the lowest aluminum brand of DTaP are used) to a whopping 1225 micrograms if the highest aluminum brands are used and a hep B vaccine is also given. Even using the large combo vaccines doesn't prevent aluminum overload. These doses are repeated at four and six months. A child would continue to get some aluminum throughout the first two years with most rounds of shots.

Just to remind you, the FDA asserts that premature babies and any patient with impaired kidney function shouldn't get more than 10 to 25 micrograms of injected aluminum at any one time.

My first instinct as a medical doctor is to worry that these aluminum levels far exceed what may be safe for young babies. But my second instinct is to assume that this issue has been researched and that studies have been done on healthy infants to determine their ability to excrete aluminum rapidly. My third instinct is to look for these studies, and so far I have not been able to find any. It is likely that the FDA thinks that the kidneys of healthy infants work well enough to excrete this aluminum rapidly before it can circulate through the body, accumulate in the brain, and cause toxic effects. However, I can't find any references in the FDA documents that show that using aluminum in vaccines has been tested and found to be safe.

So I did what any pediatrician would do. I turned to the American Academy of Pediatrics, which published a policy in 1996 called "Aluminum Toxicity in Infants and Children" (see "Resources," page 250). Here are several keys items:

- Aluminum can cause neurologic harm.

- A study from thirty years ago showed that human adults will increase their urine excretion of aluminum when exposed to higher levels (suggesting adults can clear out excess aluminum).

- Adults taking aluminum-containing antacids don't build up high levels in their body.

- There have been reports of infants with healthy kidneys showing elevated blood levels of aluminum from taking antacids.

- People with kidney disease who build up levels of aluminum greater than 100 micrograms per liter in their bloodstream are at risk for toxicity.

- The toxic threshold may be even lower.

- Aluminum loading (tissue buildup) has been seen even in patients with healthy kidneys who receive IV solutions containing aluminum over extended periods.

Completely absent from this paper was any mention whatsoever of aluminum in vaccines.

To put this information in perspective, an average adult has about 5 liters of blood. So having more than 500 micrograms in the bloodstream all at once would be toxic if his kidneys weren't working well. Toxicity has also been seen in patients with healthy kidneys. A newborn has a blood volume of about a third of a liter, or 300 milliliters. So having more than 30 micrograms floating around in his bloodstream at once could be toxic if the baby's kidneys weren't working well. A child has about 1 liter of blood, so more than 100 micrograms in his system could be toxic. I've already stated that babies are sometimes injected with more than 100 micrograms at one time. Fortunately, this amount doesn't go into the bloodstream all at once. It's slowly diffused into the bloodstream over a period of time from the muscle or skin where it is injected.

But that is my main point. No one has ever measured the levels of aluminum absorption into the bloodstream, then excretion into the urine and out of the body, when it is injected into the skin and muscle of infants. All the FDA and AAP documents say is that it may be a problem, but we haven't studied it yet, so we should limit aluminum in injectable solutions. But no one is talking about the levels in vaccines.

What I think may have happened is that aluminum used to be in only one vaccine (DTP), so no one thought much about it. Then along came the PedVaxHIB brand of HIB vaccine in the 1980s; PedVaxHIB contains aluminum, but the other brands of HIB vaccine did not, so no one thought much about it. Then we started using the hep B vaccine in the 1990s, the Pc vaccine in the 2000s, and recently the hep A and HPV vaccines. Giving one aluminum vaccine at a time doesn't amount to much aluminum, but giving four together really adds up. It seems that this issue has simply escaped everyone's attention. Or has it?

Researchers from the Cochrane Collaboration (a group that looks at health care issues around the world) investigated aluminum in vaccines and published its findings in *The Lancet: Infectious Diseases* in 2004 (see "Resources," page 250). This group reviewed all the side effect testing for one particular aluminum-containing vaccine (DTP) and looked for any evidence that it caused more side effects than nonaluminum vaccines. Other than more redness, swelling, and pain at the injection site, the Cochrane Collaboration didn't find any indications that an aluminum-containing vaccine caused any problems. What prompted the investigation? According to *The Lancet* journal, there have been suspected cases of aluminum causing various neurologic and degenerative problems. The Cochrane Collaboration wanted to look at a very large study group to see if there was a real correlation. It didn't find any problems with aluminum in vaccines and concluded that no further research should be undertaken on this topic.

That's a pretty bold statement. Most researchers will make a conclusion on research findings, but it's unusual to go so far as to say that no one else should do any more research into the matter.

What's more, the Cochrane Collaboration didn't actually study aluminum metabolism itself. It didn't test aluminum levels in kids after vaccination. It didn't explore whether or not the amount of aluminum in vaccines builds up in the brain or bone tissues. It just looked for evidence of visible symptoms of toxicity, without even looking for internal aluminum effects. And it didn't do its own research. It simply reviewed all available studies done by others. Also, it looked only at one aluminum-containing vaccine instead of testing all four at once. The Cochrane Collaboration essentially closed the book on aluminum without ever really opening it.

The most obvious way to study this matter would be to inject various amounts of aluminum into kids to see what happens to it internally. We know from the FDA documents that aluminum toxicity does occur from other types of injectable treatments, that it accumulates in the brain and bones in toxic amounts, that this toxicity may occur more commonly than is recognized, and that it's hard to detect just by observing symptoms. So what happens when the amount of aluminum contained in vaccines is injected?

I think vaccine manufacturers may have started wondering the same thing, because I found some interesting research in the product insert of the brand-new HPV vaccine. Merck actually added a little extra step to its safety research by injecting aluminum into a separate group of test subjects to use as a safety control group. It studied some of the side effects of the new vaccine compared to a saline placebo as well as the aluminum placebo. Merck found that the placebo with aluminum was a lot more painful than the saline placebo, and just about as painful as the full HPV shot. The aluminum placebo also caused a lot more redness, swelling, and itching than the saline placebo, but not quite as much as the full HPV shot. Unfortunately, Merck looked only at aluminum effects right at the injection site. It didn't state in the product insert what role the aluminum placebo played in all the other standard side effects like fever and flu-like symptoms, although it probably has these data. And it didn't study internal aluminum metabolism. But this research did show how reactive aluminum can be when injected into the muscles, and it was a good first step. I'm hoping that someone who is research-minded and curious about this issue will explore it in complete detail so I can put it behind me, and you can feel more confident about vaccine safety. I will post any new developments about aluminum on www.TheVaccineBook.com.

Because aluminum may be toxic, why not just take it out of the vaccines, as was done with mercury? The problem is, aluminum is an adjuvant. This means that it helps the vaccines to work better. When aluminum is mixed with the vaccine components, the body's immune system recognizes the vaccines better. So to take it out would decrease the vaccine's effectiveness. The Cochrane Collaboration also pointed out that removing aluminum from vaccines would be a huge undertaking, requiring extensive trials of reformulated vaccines.

Mercury was easy to take out, because it had nothing to do with helping the vaccine work. But the pharmaceutical companies would need to have some good evidence that aluminum is harmful before they would invest in reformulating vaccines without aluminum.

What exactly does aluminum do in the brain when it builds up in toxic amounts? While no one has studied healthy babies to see how much, if any, aluminum from vaccines builds up, the study on IV feeding solutions in premature babies I discussed on page 196 revealed that aluminum impaired their neurologic and mental development (see "Resources," page 251). But that was in premature babies, not full-term healthy ones. I found several animal studies involving aluminum and/or aluminum-containing vaccines that did show neurologic harm (see "Resources," page 252). The aluminum built up in the brain and caused damage, some of which looked similar to what is seen in the brains of Alzheimer's patients. But it's hard to correlate these findings precisely into human terms. What we need are more human infant studies.

Parents who wish to be very cautious and limit their baby's exposure to aluminum can do the following:

- Ask your doctor to order the brand of HIB vaccine that does not contain aluminum (see page 6).

- Ask your doctor to avoid the brand of DTaP with the most amount of aluminum (see page 34). However, you should be aware that the DTaP with the lowest aluminum also has a trace of mercury and uses cow tissue in manufacturing. The brand of DTaP with a moderate amount of aluminum does *not* contain mercury and does *not* use cow tissues.

- As for the hepatitis B, Pc, hepatitis A, and HPV vaccines, all available brands have the same amount of aluminum. Parents can limit the number of aluminum-containing vaccines given at any one time, but then their children will have to come in for extra "shot only" visits between checkups. In chapter 19, "What Should You Now Do?," I will detail a vaccine schedule that allows you to get every vaccine in a timely manner, while getting only one aluminum-containing vaccine at a time.

- Avoid any combo vaccines that have more aluminum than the individual shots do (see page 198).

If I could sum up the aluminum controversy in three sentences, it would be this: There is good evidence that large amounts of aluminum *are* harmful to humans. There is no solid evidence that the amount of aluminum in vaccines is harmful to infants and children. No one has actually studied vaccine amounts of aluminum in healthy human infants to make sure it is safe. Should we now stop and research this matter? Or should we just go on and continue to hope that it is safe?

Vaccine policymakers and advocates who read my concerns about aluminum will probably initiate several research studies to explore its risks. But I hope they won't conduct a simple retrospective review of all the old vaccine safety studies and journal articles to look for aluminum side effects. Because they won't find any. Aluminum toxicity, as the FDA, AAP, and others have stated, can't be noticed just by external observation. It would really be a shame to find several such reports show up in the medical literature trying to put a lid on this issue. The only way to put it to rest is for someone to conduct several real-time studies on thousands of human infants and measure aluminum levels after vaccination. And researchers should look not just at blood levels. They should find out where aluminum accumulates in the body, if at all; how it is eliminated from the body; and at what rate. Once I see such research, and I determine to my satisfaction that aluminum has been proven safe, then I will post an update on www.TheVaccineBook.com and revise this section of the book for the next edition. If we find that aluminum may not be safe, then I would expect a new vaccine schedule to be adopted that spaces out the aluminum vaccines (see page 223 for such a schedule). I would also expect vaccine manufacturers to find ways to reduce or remove aluminum from vaccines without compromising their effectiveness. One brand of the HIB vaccine requires aluminum to make it work, but another brand doesn't. One brand of DTaP has four times as much aluminum as another brand. Some vaccines don't have any aluminum at all. So we already know that vaccines can work without aluminum or with reduced amounts.

I worry that aluminum may end up being another thimerosal (mercury). I know that research has not been able to prove that the mercury in vaccines is harmful, and I am relieved that it has been taken out of most vaccines as of 2002. But according to an article in the *Los Angeles Times* on February 8, 2005, Merck knew in 1991 that the cumulative amount of mercury in vaccines given to infants by six months of age was about eighty-seven times what was thought to be safe. If you've never read that article, I encourage you to do so. It shows a copy of an internal memo written by one of Merck's research doctors and sent to the president of Merck's vaccine division. The memo clearly states the worry about mercury overload. What was done with that information back in 1991? We'll never know. What we do know is that vaccine manufacturers knew we were overdosing babies with mercury, but no one in the medical community realized the possible implications for almost ten years. Why? Because no one talked about it. When we did find out, we hoped it wasn't harmful, we did extensive research to show it wasn't harmful, and we slowly removed it from most vaccines. And now the point is moot for infants getting vaccines today.

But what isn't moot is the question of aluminum. Doctors can choose certain vaccine brands that have less or no aluminum. We can be careful about giving only one aluminum-containing vaccine at a time. And we can talk about it instead of brushing the issue under the carpet. I pray that my fears about aluminum are unfounded, and that several unbiased, objective studies done by completely independent groups who have no ties to vaccine manufacturers or political organizations show that aluminum is safe. If not, I hope that vaccine manufacturers will start to reduce aluminum as soon as possible. The task won't be easy, but our children are worth it.

OTHER CHEMICAL ADDITIVES

One common criticism of vaccines is that they contain many unusual ingredients and chemicals. Some people worry that these chemicals aren't all safe. Fortunately they are administered in such tiny amounts that our bodies should be able to process and eliminate them without harm. Most of these chemicals have gone through extensive animal testing. Some have been shown to be okay while others are known toxins and carcinogens. Many haven't been adequately tested in humans. No one has ever examined the toxic effects of these chemicals by injecting the amounts used in vaccines into babies and then doing blood and tissue evaluations to look for toxic effects. So it would be fair to say that we don't know that every chemical used in vaccines is 100 percent safe. To go into detail on the toxicology of each chemical is beyond the scope of this book. I have included a brief summary of each chemical used in vaccines. For more details on each, you can consult a variety of online chemical databases.

Mercury

Mercury, or thimerosal, has been a very hot topic in the medical and political arena for the past several years. It seems as if anyone who even tries to question why mercury used to be in vaccines is immediately shot down by a barrage of medical experts and politicians claiming that there is no evidence that mercury causes any harm. We know the rate of autism has increased dramatically over the past decade or so. Several studies have shown no correlation between mercury in vaccines and the rise of neurologic diseases like autism. Some studies do show a rise in autism starting when the number of vaccines containing mercury was increased in the early 1990s, as well as a decrease in the past few years now that mercury has been removed from vaccines (see "Resources," page 260).

So who do we believe? Fortunately for those of you deciding about vaccines right now, the only vaccines in which mercury is even an issue are some brands of the flu shot and some tetanus shots. Finding a mercury-free flu shot can be quite a challenge, however. Every year, manufacturers make only a limited supply of flu shots without mercury. It's much easier to make larger batches of the vaccine in 10-dose bottles with mercury as a preservative in order to meet the demands of our population. But other than this, you can get the entire vaccine schedule mercury free. So you don't even have to figure out who is right and wrong. Just make sure your doctor uses mercury-free flu shots.

Now, what about those shots that contain traces of mercury? This amount is about 1/100 of what it used to be, so I consider it too negligible to worry about. But if you want to worry anyway, you can ask your doctor for a completely mercury-free brand. Here is a list of the current vaccines that contain a trace amount of mercury:

- Tripedia brand of DTaP
- Plain tetanus in the single-dose vial
- DT in the single-dose vial
- dT in the single-dose vial
- Fluarix and Fluvirin brands of flu shot

The following shots are the only ones (as of the writing of this book) that contain a full 25-microgram dose of mercury:

- Plain tetanus in the multidose vial
- dT in the multidose vial
- DT in the multidose vial (no longer produced, but old bottles may still be out there)
- Fluzone and FluLaval brands of the flu shot in a multidose vial (Fluzone's single-dose vial does not have any mercury)

Do I think mercury is harmful? Yes. Do I think the amount in the old vaccines caused harm? I'm not 100 percent convinced one way or the other. I think no one has proven that it was safe, and the studies showing some harmful effects from vaccines containing mercury are thought-provoking. But the good news is that I don't have to decide, and neither do you. Mercury is now, for the most part, a thing of the past.

Formaldehyde

This chemical preserved the frogs, cats, or whatever types of cadavers you dissected in biology class. It is present in several vaccines in very tiny amounts as a preservative. The Environmental Protection Agency, Occupational Safety and Health Administration, Consumer Product Safety Commission, and other agencies all list formaldehyde as a carcinogen and state that it can cause kidney damage and genetic damage. Most of the research on formaldehyde, however, deals with inhaled levels of the chemical. I could not find information on injected formaldehyde. Fortunately, the amount in each vaccine is minuscule.

Polysorbate 80 and 20

These chemicals are present in a number of products and foods, not just vaccines. They have been tested and are generally regarded as safe.

MSG

Monosodium glutamate is in some vaccines. This flavor enhancer used in many different foods has been the subject of heated debate for years. Some studies show that MSG is considered an excitotoxin (a chemical that can affect how the brain functions) and that when consumed in large quantities or injected into the brains of animals it can damage nerve tissue in a pattern similar to Alzheimer's disease. Because of such concerns, MSG has been removed from many products, including baby food. Fortunately, the amount of MSG in vaccines is about half a milligram. The amount consumed in a serving of Chinese food, just for comparison, is between 1000 and 10,000 milligrams. See "Resources," page 268.

EDTA

This chemical is used in a variety of consumer products. It is also used as a heavy-metal detoxifier in lead-poisoning patients. The tiny amount in some vaccines is negligible and considered harmless.

2-Phenoxyethanol

This chemical is used as a preservative. Researchers have found that it is harmful if swallowed, inhaled, or absorbed through the skin; it may cause reproductive defects and is severely irritating to the eyes and skin. It is also used in perfumes and cosmetics, insect repellents, antiseptics, plasticizers, germicides, pharmaceuticals, preservatives, and as a solvent for dyes, inks, and resins. Even though 2-phenoxyethanol seems fairly toxic, the amount in vaccines is minuscule.

Sodium borate

Sodium borate is used to decrease acidity in vaccines. It is considered harmless.

Octoxynol

This chemical is used as a spermacide in other products. The tiny amount in vaccines is considered harmless.

Sodium deoxycholate

This chemical is harmful if swallowed, inhaled, or absorbed through the skin and can irritate the eyes and lungs. The amount in vaccines is minuscule.

Fortunately, all of these chemicals, even the toxic ones, are used in very tiny amounts in vaccines. Our bodies should be able to handle them. It would be more reassuring, however, if we had better studies on precise toxicology in human infants. Anyone want to volunteer your baby? Very cautious parents may choose to get fewer vaccines at a time in order to spread out exposure to chemicals.

17

Myths and Questions
about Vaccines

ARE VACCINES 100 PERCENT EFFECTIVE?

No, they are not. Very few vaccines have ever claimed to work 100 percent of the time. (The tetanus vaccine *is* thought to be completely effective.) Vaccine efficacy varies, but in general most vaccines are about 85 to 95 percent effective in preventing disease. Some vaccine opponents use this fact to argue against vaccination. ("Aha! The vaccine isn't 100 percent protective!") But even though they aren't perfect, vaccines still offer very good protection. If a roomful of a hundred vaccinated kids is exposed to a disease, only about ten of the kids will catch that illness. Compare that to a roomful of unvaccinated kids. Most of them will come down with the disease and spread it to other kids. An added perk for vaccinated kids is that any disease they do catch will likely run a milder course.

HOW DO VACCINES WORK?

Vaccines work by fooling the body's immune system into thinking that the disease is attacking. When a live virus, inactivated whole-cell bacteria, or just portions of a germ are injected or swallowed in a vaccine, the immune cells recognize it as the disease and create an immune response. This immunity is "remembered" for many years. So if the real disease ever invades, the immune system is ready with an immediate response, thus preventing the disease or making it less severe.

HOW LONG DO VACCINES LAST?

Most vaccines last about ten to fifteen years. But there are two aspects to this issue. Detectable antibody levels in the blood from a particular vaccine may last ten years, yet the body's immune system may still retain some protection even after the blood antibody levels diminish. No researcher has been able to clearly determine how long each vaccine lasts, so I can't give you an exact breakdown. Suffice it to say, most infant and childhood vaccines will protect a child into the teenage years, but probably not much beyond that.

WEREN'T DISEASES ALREADY DISAPPEARING BEFORE VACCINES WERE INTRODUCED?

This is a common misconception spread by vaccine opponents. When I go to anti-vaccine lectures or read anti-vaccine books, I see diagrams showing how each disease was already disappearing before we even started using its vaccine. People claim that better health care and cleaner living standards have been responsible for eliminating most diseases and that these diseases would have eventually disappeared without the vaccines. But when I look at the data in medical books, it seems pretty clear to me that in most cases vaccines were largely responsible for eliminating or greatly reducing these diseases in the United States.

When you look at the year each vaccine was introduced (pertussis in the 1940s, polio in the 1950s, measles and rubella in the 1960s, HIB in the 1980s, and chickenpox in the 1990s, just to name a few examples) and when each disease quickly declined to low levels in our population, it is obvious that the vaccine played a major role. Sure, some diseases were already *declining* before a vaccine was widely administered, but without the actual vaccines most diseases would have continued at much higher levels than they are at today. In fact, most vaccine-preventable diseases have nothing to do with poor health care or unsanitary living conditions. They can easily spread among the cleanest and healthiest of people. Even *my* wife caught whooping cough a few years ago. And she takes a shower *almost* every day.

SHOULD PAIN-RELIEVING MEDICATIONS BE GIVEN BEFORE SHOTS?

One way to minimize uncomfortable reactions to vaccines is to give your child ibuprofen about thirty minutes prior to the shots (acetaminophen can also be used, although it may be less effective; ibuprofen isn't approved until three months of age). Bring some with you to the doctor's office and give it to your child when the nurse first puts you into an exam room for your checkup. In waiting for the doctor, having your checkup, then sitting around to wait for shots, you can be sure that at least a half hour will have passed.

I am not a big fan of premedicating. It can mask the outward symptoms of an internal reaction. If a baby is going to react to a vaccine with three days of high fever and high-pitched screaming, you and the doctor should know this in order to decide how to approach subsequent vaccines. If these symptoms are covered up, you will never know that your baby's brain and body are reacting poorly. Once you get to know how your baby reacts after one or two rounds of a particular vaccine, and you've seen some mild but tolerable reactions, you and your doctor can decide about premedicating for the rest of the shots.

IS THERE ANY WAY TO TAKE THE STING OUT OF SHOTS?

Parents can apply an over-the-counter numbing cream containing lidocaine to the injection sites about forty-five minutes prior to the shots to minimize the pain. This cream is also available by prescription. For infants in the first year, shots are given in the upper, outer portion of the thighs. After one year, they are usually given in the shoulder. You can put the cream on at home or have a nurse help you when you first get to the doctor's office before your checkup begins.

I don't usually recommend this practice. The cream is expensive, it relieves only *some* of the pain, and parents who apply it to their baby at home before their visit often don't put it in the right place. Overall, I'm not sure it's worth the cost and trouble. Instead of using cream, you can firmly rub the anticipated injection site for a few minutes prior to the shots to desensitize the area enough to decrease the pain. Rubbing ice on the area for a minute is also effective, but not exactly pleasant for a baby. Breastfeeding during a vaccination (or any painful procedure) has been shown to decrease discomfort in babies.

IS IT OKAY FOR A SICK BABY TO GET SHOTS?

It's inevitable. The day before your baby's checkup, her nose starts to run. Or she's just coming off antibiotics from an ear infection. What do you do? Some people worry that vaccines may temporarily lower a child's immune system, thus making any present illness potentially worse. Although this theory hasn't been proven in research studies, it makes sense. As the immune system is working on the vaccines, other parts of the immune system may be "distracted" or may not work at full capacity. So vaccinating may make a mild illness worse. Another complicating factor is that if the shots make your baby fussy and feverish for a couple days, you won't be able to tell whether it's her illness that's worsening or just a reaction to the vaccines. On the other hand, if you delay your baby's shots and come back a few weeks later to get the shots when she's completely well, there goes another co-pay!

The reality is that some kids are sick more often than they are well. If we waited for every child to be completely free from any illness, some kids would never get vaccinated. In general, if an illness is minor enough to allow a child into school or day care and doesn't require antibiotics, then it's probably okay to give the shots. If a child is sick enough to need antibiotics or to stay home from school, or is fussy and not sleeping or eating well, then shots should be put off until another day.

I would also recommend that the MMR vaccine not be given when a child is suffering from diarrhea or has taken antibiotics in the past few weeks. This vaccine may cause more reactions when the intestines aren't at peak health.

CATCHING UP WHEN YOU MISS DOSES
AT THE NORMALLY SCHEDULED TIME

Even though the shots are designed to be given at certain intervals, the schedule isn't set in stone. The timing can vary by many months. Some vaccines have courses of three or four shots, but doctors still have some play in determining when to give them. If you fall behind in a series of four shots, you don't have to start over again when you resume. You just pick up where you left off, even if years have gone by. I was once appalled when a school nurse told a parent in my practice that her five-year-old needed the entire hep B three-shot series all over again because she had gotten only two of the shots as a baby.

STOPPING SHOTS BEFORE A SERIES IS COMPLETE

Parents often ask me if they absolutely must complete a particular series of shots once they have started it. They worry that not finishing the series will cause problems for their child. The only downside to abandoning a series of shots in midstream is that the child won't have full protection. Other than that, a child can stop vaccines at any time without any negative effects.

ARE VACCINES REQUIRED FOR SCHOOL, CAMP, AND DAY CARE?

Public schools and public day cares "require" a child to be fully immunized for entry. However, this requirement isn't absolute. All states allow parents to waive any vaccine for medical reasons, with a note from the doctor. All states (except Mississippi and West Virginia—read on) allow parents to waive vaccines for religious reasons. Sure, the school will hassle you and give you the "bad parent" speech, but legally the administrators must let your child in. Some states require very strict proof that your religion opposes vaccines, and others don't. Twenty states—Arkansas, Arizona (read on), California, Colorado, Idaho, Louisiana, Maine, Michigan, Minnesota, New Mexico, North Dakota, Ohio, Oklahoma, Oregon, Pennsylvania, Texas, Utah, Vermont, Washington, and Wisconsin—are more lenient. They don't require you to have a medical or religious reason. You can simply waive vaccines for personal or philosophical reasons. In fact, you don't even need to provide a reason.

In Arizona the situation is a little confusing. According to my research, Arizonans must have religious reasons for waiving vaccines in day care (personal reasons don't count at that age). By the time a child enters school, his parents simply need a personal reason to waive the shots, but religious reasons are no longer valid.

There are two states that absolutely require all children to be immunized in order to enter any day care or school program: Mississippi and West Virginia. I've heard rumors that state child protective services take children away from their parents if they don't immunize. I find that hard to believe, but if you live in one of these two states and don't want to vaccinate, it might be time to move (or hide for a really long time).

(This state-by-state information comes from Johns Hopkins University, updated March 2006; see "Resources," page 267.)

Private schools and day cares are another matter. In most states, they don't have to follow the state rules on vaccines (except for Mississippi and West Virginia, where the laws apply to all schools). Private institutions can choose to be more lenient or more strict. They can deny your child admission if he isn't vaccinated. Most private schools and day cares won't go that far, but they have the legal right to do so.

If you are planning not to vaccinate your child and intend to send him to private school or day care, check the school's policy before applying. It wouldn't make sense to try to catch your child up on all his shots at age five just because the private school you happen to want to send him to requires it. No school is *that* good. Almost every city has at least one school or day-care center that is more lenient than others about its vaccine requirements.

What about camps and clubs? These organizations work the same way as private schools. They can deny your child entrance into their program if they so choose.

Understand that these vaccine requirements simply mean that your child must be vaccinated by the time you enroll him into a program that will check vaccine records. You don't have to overload your baby with vaccines right from the start just so you can enroll him in school five years later. Also, if you don't vaccinate your child in the early years, but need to vaccinate him for school entry, you don't need to catch up on all the shots. The exact requirements vary from state to state, and your public school will give you specific information for your state. But in general, if you don't start any vaccines until age three or later, you won't need HIB, Pc, or rotavirus. The flu vaccine usually isn't required for school entry. Hep A vaccine requirements vary, and you will need both shots if it is mandatory. But you may need only three DTaPs instead of five. You may need only three polios instead of four. You may need only one MMR and chickenpox if they are given after age four. You will probably need all three hep Bs. The twelve-year shot requirements (Tdap, meningococcal, and HPV) vary from state to state, but this schedule doesn't affect your decision at kindergarten entry. See chapter 18 for more information on catching up on vaccines that you delayed or skipped during your child's infancy.

IS IT YOUR SOCIAL RESPONSIBILITY TO VACCINATE YOUR KIDS?

This is one of the most controversial aspects of the vaccine debate. Obviously, the more kids who are vaccinated, the better our
country is protected and the less likely it is that any child will die
from a disease. Some parents, however, aren't willing to risk the
very rare side effects of vaccines, so they choose to skip the shots.
Their children benefit from herd immunity (the protection of all
the vaccinated kids around them) without risking the vaccines
themselves. Is this selfish? Perhaps. But as parents you have to
decide. Are you supposed to make decisions that are good for the
country as a whole? Or do you base your decision on what's best
for your own child as an individual? Can we fault parents for putting their own child's health ahead of the other kids' around him?

From a public health standpoint, we *can* find fault. Parents
who don't vaccinate increase the likelihood that diseases will
spread through our population and put the rest of us at risk. If
you ask Spock, second in command of the starship *Enterprise,*
he'll tell you, "The needs of the many outweigh the needs of the
few . . . or the one." However, Spock made this comment as he
was in the process of dying to save the whole crew. Would his
mom think her son had made the right choice? Maybe. But I'm
sure she wasn't thrilled to hear about his death. And she didn't
have the benefit of knowing he would come back to life in the
very next movie. (I like to incorporate *Star Trek* wisdom into
most of life's important decisions.)

Now back to reality. From a freedom-of-choice point of view,
we can't really fault parents who think that vaccines are too risky
and decide to put their own kids first. We all put our own children first in most situations. As long as we have the freedom to
choose what's best for our own kids, parents will, and should,
continue to have the right to decline vaccination.

I've always been fascinated with the reasons parents choose to take a chance with the diseases instead of risk the vaccines (which statistically seem less risky). One patient summed it up in a very interesting way that I'd never thought about. She said that if she chose to vaccinate her children, she would be actively taking a risk. She would be purposely deciding to take that 1 in 2600 chance. If one of her kids suffered a bad side effect, it would be because of something she did. If, on the other hand, she didn't vaccinate, she would be taking a passive risk; she would be taking the chance that something (a disease) would *not* happen to her kids. She's leaving it up to nature, or chance, or God. If her children suffer a severe course of a disease, it won't be because of something she did. Rather, it will be because of something she didn't do. She said she would rather live with that type of choice.

18

Parents Who Delay or Decline Vaccination

A small percentage of parents ultimately choose to delay vaccines or decline them altogether. Although that idea runs contrary to the thinking of most doctors, I understand that many of these parents are really set on their decision. I generally don't try too hard to talk these parents out of their choice, but I do like to offer them a little bit of advice, and I offer it to you now.

Although some of the vaccines you are skipping are for mild diseases, others are designed to prevent potentially life-threatening illnesses. So I want to make sure you know what vaccines are the most important ones that you may want to reconsider giving. I call this approach "Selective Vaccination": giving your child the most crucial shots at the age when they are most needed, and skipping or delaying the less critical shots (which you were already going to say no to anyway). This Selective Vaccination Schedule is what I tell parents to consider when they otherwise would have declined all vaccines. Here are the criteria I use to decide which vaccines are the most important:

1. The disease is likely to be very severe (fatal, permanently disabling, or requiring hospitalization).

Dr. Bob's
Selective Vaccination Schedule

2 months	DTaP, Rotavirus
3 months	Pc, HIB
4 months	DTaP, Rotavirus
5 months	Pc, HIB
6 months	DTaP, Rotavirus
7 months	Pc, HIB
15 months	Pc, HIB
5 years	Tetanus booster
10 years	Blood tests for measles, mumps, rubella, chickenpox, and hep A immunity (see page 227). Consider vaccinating if not immune. Also consider a 3-dose polio series if travel to Africa or Asia is a possibility.
11 years	HPV (3 doses, girls only). See my note in the next section.
12 years	Hep B (3 doses)

2. The disease is not only severe, it's also fairly common.
3. The vaccines have the lowest probability of causing a severe reaction and have as few controversial ingredients as possible.

My Selective Vaccination Schedule leaves out the shots that tend to have more severe or more frequent side effects. It omits vaccines for diseases that are usually mild, don't occur during young childhood, don't exist in our country, or are fairly rare. Although these shots are still important for the immunity of our nation as a whole, they just don't fit all the criteria choosy parents have. The shots I've listed fit at least two of my three criteria.

WHY THESE SHOTS?

DTaP. Although diphtheria and tetanus don't fit my criteria, pertussis certainly does. It's common, it's potentially severe in the first year of life, and the side effect profile of the vaccine is acceptable. The ingredients do include some chemicals, but overall it fits most of the criteria. The eighteen-month DTaP that is normally recommended isn't as critical after the first year of life, so I don't include it here. The tetanus booster is shown at age five to provide protection for the growing child.

Rotavirus. Rotavirus is certainly common, potentially severe for infants, and the ingredients and known side effects of the vaccine so far are reasonable.

Pc. *Pneumococcus* is a very common germ, yet most cases are fairly mild. Severe cases of Pc are uncommon but do occur. The side effects and ingredients of the vaccine are acceptable.

HIB. HIB is a severe disease when it does strike, but fortunately it is extremely rare now. The ingredients and side effects of the vaccine seem to be among the safest of all shots.

HPV. HPV is an important disease to try to prevent, but the vaccine is too new for me to sign off on completely. If the safety and effectiveness of the HPV vaccine pan out over the next couple of years, then I will probably keep it on my list. Visit www.TheVaccineBook.com for updates.

Hep B. Although hepatitis B is very severe when it occurs in babies and children, it is rare in that age group and the listed vaccine side effects do include some potentially bad reactions, so I didn't put it on my list for infants. I do, however, put it on the list for preteens.

It's important to note that I recommend most of these shots be given during the ages when they are most needed—infancy for the first four vaccines and the preteen years for the last two. It wouldn't make much sense to wait until age one or two to give the infant shots because the child is way past the age when these illnesses tend to strike and strike hard. I also realize that parents who do not wish to vaccinate think their kids don't need hep B or HPV protection until the teen years (or never at all for those with perfect children), so I don't push until the shots become more relevant.

So, parents who are thinking of not getting any vaccines for their children, please consider the shots in my Selective Vaccination Schedule. You will notice that it calls for only two shots at a time and only one aluminum-containing vaccine at a time. It protects your baby from diseases that could be fatal without overloading him with shots.

What about all the other shots? Aren't they important too? Yes, they are, but they don't fit most of the criteria I use for Selective Vaccination for parents who otherwise weren't going to vaccinate. Here are my reasons for not including the rest of the shots:

Polio. This disease doesn't occur in the United States, and its ingredients include more chemicals than most vaccines as well as some blood products (although the side effects of the shot seem mild).

Flu. Because of some of the ingredients and the high percentage of reactions from this vaccine, I don't put it on the list. Although it is a very common illness, and it does cause many hospitalizations, infant and child fatalities are rare.

MMR. For the most part, measles, mumps, and rubella are (or used to be) routine childhood illnesses with very few problems. These diseases are now fairly rare. And the side effect profile of the vaccine is the longest and most potentially severe (although rare) of all the shots.

Chickenpox. Although still very common, this illness is usually mild. There are some notable side effects from and unusual ingredients in the vaccine that worry choosy parents.

Hepatitis A. This disease is somewhat common, but most childhood cases are mild. The vaccine ingredients do include some chemicals and unusual components, and the potential seizure side effect is also something to consider.

Meningococcal vaccine. A severe disease, but it's fairly uncommon. The ingredients of this vaccine are safe, but the very rare side effect of Guillan-Barré syndrome is something to consider. Also, I don't include this vaccine on the list because it is so new. If the safety profile continues to look good after several years, I may add this vaccine to the selective list for teenagers. Once it is found to be safe and effective and approved for younger children, I may eventually add it to the selective list at age two. Watch www.TheVaccineBook.com for updates.

GETTING A BLOOD TEST TO DETERMINE
WHETHER A SHOT IS NEEDED

Children can get a blood test (called a "titer") before getting a vaccine to see if they happened to be exposed to the disease enough during childhood to acquire immunity. If a titer is positive, the child may not need the shot. Parents who skip the chickenpox vaccine, for example, will usually get their kids tested during the preteen years, then consider getting the shot if the test shows no immunity. Titer testing is available for almost all diseases, but it is more accurate for the *viral* illnesses like measles, mumps, rubella, chickenpox, and hepatitis A. Polio, hepatitis B, and tetanus are also diseases that titers can test for, but realistically infants in the United States aren't exposed, so testing usually isn't done. Rotavirus, flu, and HPV don't have titer tests that are commercially useful.

The *bacterial* infections (HIB, Pc, diphtheria, pertussis, and *Meningococcus*) have titer tests, but we don't really know whether a positive titer for a bacterial disease indicates adequate immunity. So we don't usually test for these bacteria.

DELAYING VACCINES UNTIL AGE TWO

Parents occasionally tell me they want to wait until their child is two years old to start vaccinations. They claim that this delay allows the immune system and nervous system to mature and handle the vaccines better. I don't know if this is true because it hasn't been established by research. And remember that some of these diseases, such as HIB and *Pneumococcus,* occur mainly during infancy. Others, such as pertussis and rotavirus, are serious only during the first year or two of life. So if a person waits until a child is two to vaccinate, the child will be past the age at which these particular vaccines are most useful. Sure, these diseases can occur beyond age two, but they are either much less common or are better tolerated.

If you are so worried about vaccines that you don't get any for your child by age two, it doesn't make much sense to then go ahead and catch up with all the shots. The way I see it, you either get your baby vaccinated against the serious infant diseases (HIB, Pc, pertussis, rotavirus) *during* infancy, when they are needed, or you just skip those shots altogether. There are other vaccines that are worth considering as your child gets older. I simply want to point out the logical timing of these four infant vaccines.

DELAYING VACCINES UNTIL SIX MONTHS OR ONE YEAR

This choice is one that some parents make, usually for the same reasons as those who wait until two years. They just don't feel as comfortable leaving their child unvaccinated as long. If you've chosen to delay shots, whether it's for six months, one year, or more, you should be aware that your child would not need the entire vaccine series when you do eventually start. Your doctor can help you decide how many of each shot your child's situation calls for. But here are some general guidelines for those of you who don't start shots until six months or one year:

- For the DTaP vaccine, you would need only 3 doses of the initial 4-dose series. You would continue with the five-year and twelve-year boosters.

- For the polysaccharide vaccines, HIB and Pc, you would need 3 doses if starting between six months and twelve months, 2 doses if starting between twelve and eighteen months, and only 1 dose if you don't get any until after eighteen months.

- For protection against hepatitis B and polio, you would need all 3 doses to be fully vaccinated, even if you didn't start until later.

- Those of you who don't start the rotavirus vaccine right away, by three months of age, miss the window of opportunity for this protection. You can't start the series after three months. This might change; look for an update at www.TheVaccineBook.com.

IF YOU DON'T VACCINATE YOUR CHILDREN IN THE EARLY YEARS, WHAT DISEASES DO YOU NEED TO WORRY ABOUT AS THEY GET OLDER?

Whether you decide to delay all vaccines, or go ahead with some of the most important infant shots but delay other less critical ones, you will continually be faced with the decision of whether, eventually, to have your child get the vaccines he skipped. How do you decide which ones to do and when?

Some parents choose to skip or delay the vaccines for diseases that used to be considered routine childhood illnesses, like chickenpox, measles, mumps, rubella, and hepatitis A. Because these illnesses are usually mild during childhood, nonvaccinating parents usually don't consider these shots until their kids are teenagers (when the diseases can become more severe). Of course, if your child actually does catch one of these illnesses (and it is confirmed by a doctor), then he likely has lifetime immunity and no shot is needed. But the illnesses are fairly rare and it's unlikely that your child will catch them, so you can get a titer blood test (see page 227) to see if your child has gained immunity through exposure to the disease. Consider vaccinating if his blood test shows he doesn't have immunity.

Some parents may have skipped certain shots for illnesses that are very rare during early childhood, such as hepatitis B and tetanus. Well, these diseases become more common as a child enters the teen years, and they are serious no matter when they hit, so you may want to reconsider as your child approaches the double digits. The meningococcal and HPV vaccines (not yet offered during infancy) become part of the equation in the teenage years. Titer blood testing isn't as reliable for these germs (hep B, tetanus, *Meningococcus,* HPV), so you can't really use that option to help you decide if your teen should get these shots. You may also want to consider the polio vaccine for your older kids (if they skipped it during the early years) when international travel becomes more common.

For the live-virus vaccines, MMR and chickenpox, only 1 dose is needed for adequate immunity if you delay them until age four. Some states require 2 shots of each, regardless of when you get them. And for chickenpox, if you wait too long (until age thirteen or later) you actually need 2 doses (one to two months apart) for the vaccine to work well.

For all other vaccines that you may have skipped but now want to catch your child up on, you need the entire series—3 doses each of polio, hep B, HPV, and tetanus (any DTaPs done in the past count toward these 3 tetanus shots), 2 doses of hep A, and 1 of meningococcal vaccine.

At what age should you get your child the tetanus series if you skipped it during infancy? Virtually all cases of tetanus in the United States occur after age five, so you could probably wait until at least that age to start the series.

PRECAUTIONS TO TAKE IF YOU DON'T VACCINATE

If you don't vaccinate your kids, here are some ways you can minimize their chance of catching one of these illnesses:

Ensure a healthy immune system. Review the recommendations on pages 187 to 190 to make sure your child's immune system is at its peak.

Breastfeed for at least one year. Two is better. Formula feeding greatly increases a baby's risk of not only catching an illness, but of having a more severe course. See page 20 for more information.

Avoid nurseries for at least two years. This includes group day care as well as church and health club nurseries. Avoid large playgroups with multiple infants. Small groups with just a few other kids are probably fine, as long as no one has a cold, cough, or fever.

Seek medical care early. If your child does come down with a cough, fever, rash, or any of the specific symptoms described in this book, see your doctor right away. In many cases, early treatment for these diseases makes a big difference.

Responsibly quarantine your children if they get sick. Many vaccine-preventable diseases are hard to recognize early in the illness. For example, by the time you know your child has whooping cough he's likely to have been contagious for weeks. If your child has a bad cough, discuss the possibility of whooping cough with your doctor and keep your child home until you are sure that's not the diagnosis. Another common example is chickenpox. Many kids go to school during the first day of the illness because no one notices the first few spots. If your child has a fever, don't give her a fever reducer and send her off to school. Check her over for spots or a rash. If she has an unusual rash, keep her home until you can identify it and determine that it isn't contagious.

IF YOU DON'T VACCINATE, WHICH DISEASES ARE THE MOST WORRISOME WHEN YOU TRAVEL INTERNATIONALLY?

You may think that your child is safe here in the United States, but travel outside of North America could put your unvaccinated child at risk for catching a vaccine-preventable disease. While most of these diseases may not be severe, there are two that don't occur in the United States but may be prevalent in other countries and are potentially very severe:

Polio. This disease still occurs in areas of Asia and Africa. Before taking your unvaccinated kids to a country where contact with a polio carrier is a possibility, consider getting the three-shot series. You should start it about six months before travel. See page 78 for more details.

Diphtheria. This severe respiratory disease has a 10 percent mortality rate. It still occurs with some frequency in parts of Asia, the South Pacific, Africa, the Middle East, Central and South America, and eastern Europe. Consider a three-shot series of a diphtheria vaccine (DT, dT, DTaP, or Tdap) starting about eight months before travel. See page 39 for more information.

Not all international travel is risky. Review the travel information on page 10 to understand what type of travel may put your kids at risk.

HOW CAN YOU FIND A DOCTOR TO SERVE YOU EVEN IF YOU DON'T WANT TO VACCINATE?

I know there are many parents out there who don't want to vaccinate their children, or want to partially vaccinate, but can't find a doctor to serve them. I am creating a section on www.TheVac cineBook.com specifically devoted to this issue. Any doctors who feel comfortable having patients who don't want to follow the standard vaccine schedule can list their medical practice on my Web site by city and state. Parents can then find a doctor close to them who is open to accepting their children as patients.

19

What Should You Now Do?

I'm sure you are trying to answer the question that is on every parent's mind: What should I now do? How do you make the right choice for your child? I have offered you all the information you need to make this decision, but I have held back from actually telling you what to do. I want you to formulate your own decision without letting my opinion sway you one way or the other. I know the challenge is daunting. I have asked hundreds of parents what their conclusions are after reading this book, and I've gotten basically two answers: They tell me they were able to process this information and can now confidently make a vaccine plan for their child, or they tell me that there is simply too much to think about and they are still lost. This first group of parents is happy I didn't make it easy for them. They wanted a lot of information, and they think I gave them enough. But if you are in this second group, and you're still confused, I have good news for you. I am now going to give you a bit of assistance. I'm going to shed a little light on the subject. I've found that some of you want that extra guidance. I don't want you to finish this book and still feel lost.

Most parents who are considering vaccinating their children fall into one of three categories:

1. You believe that vaccines are important enough, the diseases risky enough, the safety research adequate enough, and the possible side effects rare enough for you to trust the opinion of our nation's top medical experts (and almost every doctor in the country), and you go ahead with the full vaccine schedule for your child as it is recommended by your doctor. If this description fits you, then you are in good company. Many American families feel the way you do. I recommend that you trust your doctor's advice, and your own intuition, and go ahead with vaccination.

2. You believe that most vaccines aren't worth the risk, especially if the corresponding diseases are mild or rare. But you do worry about the severe, common diseases, so you want to pick and choose a few vaccines for your child. If you are in this group, I hope I have helped you understand what your options are. I will trust you to read and reread this book until you feel comfortable choosing which vaccines you want. You probably found chapter 18 of particular interest.

3. You believe that all the diseases are a threat, but you worry that some of the potential problems with vaccines haven't been thoroughly researched to your satisfaction. You want to vaccinate, but you want to do so in a way that minimizes each potential risk (whether or not the risk is real). This group used to be somewhat smaller, but it has been growing in recent years as the media and the Internet bring theoretical problems with vaccines to light. Your biggest challenge is that your baby is young, you need to start vaccinating, but you just aren't sure what to do. Even though I have offered you virtually every possible detail about vaccines, I haven't been able to give you definitive information on some of their potential problems be-

Dr. Bob's
Alternative Vaccine Schedule

2 months	DTaP, Rotavirus
*3 months**	Pc, HIB
4 months	DTaP, Rotavirus
*5 months**	Pc, HIB
6 months	DTaP, Rotavirus
*7 months**	Pc, HIB
9 months	Polio, Flu (2 doses†)
12 months	Mumps, Polio
15 months	Pc, HIB
18 months	DTaP, Chickenpox

* The 3-, 5-, and 7-month vaccines occur during what I call "shot-only" visits. You don't need a full checkup every single month (unless your baby has some problems that require extra attention). These shot-only visits are scheduled with the nurse.

† The flu vaccine would start between 6 and 12 months if nearing flu season, then yearly thereafter, up to age 5, as flu season approaches. Try to use only a mercury-free shot. If it's not available, don't get it that year, or get the nasal spray.

cause I couldn't find enough medical evidence to close the book on every issue. So what should you do?

For the benefit of those of you in this third group, let's pretend for a moment that some of the potential risks of vaccines are real.

*21 months**	Flu
2 years	Rubella, Polio
*2 years, 6 months**	Hep B†, Hep A
3 years	Hep B, Measles, Flu‡
*3 years, 6 months**	Hep B, Hep A
4 years	DTaP, Polio, Flu‡
5 years	MMR§, Flu‡
6 years	Chickenpox
12 years	Tdap, HPV
*12 years, 2 months**	HPV
13 years	HPV, Meningococcal**

* The shots given at 21 months, 2½ years, 3½ years, and 12 years, 2 months are "shot-only" visits.

† Start the hep B vaccine at birth if Mom, Dad, or any close family members are hep B carriers.

‡ The flu shot is given at separate visits in October or November at ages 3, 4, and 5.

§ Even though I give the first M, M, and R separately, it may be okay to group them together into the MMR shot for the booster because an older child may handle it better. An alternative choice would be to give the M, M, and R boosters separately over a few years again, starting at age 5.

** Once the meningococcal vaccine is approved for age 2, I'll move it there and delay hep B by 6 months.

How would one go about fully vaccinating while avoiding these risks? Is that even possible? I believe it is. I have put together a vaccine schedule that gets children fully vaccinated, but does so in a way that minimizes the theoretical risks of vaccines. It's the best of both worlds of disease prevention and safe vaccination.

As a reminder, here is the American Academy of Pediatrics 2007 Recommended Vaccine Schedule:

American Academy of Pediatrics
2007 Recommended Vaccine Schedule

Birth	Hep B
1 month	Hep B
2 months	HIB, Pc, DTaP, Rotavirus, Polio
4 months	HIB, Pc, DTaP, Rotavirus, Polio
6 months	HIB, Pc, DTaP, Rotavirus, Hep B, Flu
1 year	MMR, Chickenpox, Hep A
15 months	HIB, Pc
18 months	DTaP, Polio, Hep A, Flu
2 years	Flu
3 years	Flu
4 years	Flu
5 years	DTaP, Polio, MMR, Flu, Chickenpox
12 years	Tdap, Meningococcal, HPV (3 doses, girls only)

As you compare the alternative schedule to the standard one recommended by the American Academy of Pediatrics, you will notice several key differences:

1. The alternative suggests only one aluminum-containing vaccine at a time in the infant years (the right brands must be chosen). By spreading out the shots, you spread out the exposure so infants can process the aluminum without it reaching toxic levels.

2. It gives no more than two vaccines at any one time to limit and spread out exposure to the numerous chemicals so a baby's system can process each more individually. Of course, we don't know whether this precaution is necessary, but it's reasonable.

3. It gives no more than two vaccines at a time to limit potential side effects. We don't know if giving six simultaneous vaccines causes more side effects, but again, giving fewer is a reasonable precaution.

4. It starts out with the most important vaccines, the ones that prevent the diseases that are most threatening to infants (DTaP, rotavirus, Pc, HIB).

5. It delays shots for diseases that are usually fairly mild for infants (hepatitis A, rubella), in order to give priority to more important shots.

6. It delays the shots for diseases that a baby is extremely unlikely to catch during the first few years of life (hepatitis B, polio) and gives them after the more important shots are almost done. By delaying some vaccines until the second or third year of life, the chemicals in these vaccines may be less likely to cause trouble; a toddler's nervous system is more mature and theoretically more able to handle chemical exposure than an infant's. In our office, we don't give the hep B vaccine to newborns. It seems

illogical to give a newborn baby a vaccine for a sexually transmitted disease (unless the mother is hep B positive). The vaccine can cause side effects that mimic the symptoms of severe
infection (fever, lethargy, poor appetite, vomiting). Newborns
who show these symptoms are hospitalized, treated with IV antibiotics, and subjected to invasive tests to rule out infection.
Why not just simply wait until a baby is a bit older, when such
side effect symptoms aren't as alarming? See "Resources" to
find a study showing how the hep B vaccine may cause more
than twice as many newborns to undergo such treatment.

7. It gives live-virus vaccines one at a time so that a baby's immune system can deal with each disease separately (rotavirus,
nasal-spray flu; separate M, M, and R; chickenpox). Splitting
the MMR into separate components is thought by some researchers to decrease the risk of autism and other reactions, although medical science has not proven that this is so. It's
probably okay to give the combination MMR booster at age
five, when a child's immune system is more mature.

8. It does not use any mercury-containing flu vaccines in infants.
It's not worth the risk.

9. It doesn't use any combination shots, which don't fit into the
schedule and can increase the simultaneous chemical exposure.

10. By giving only two shots at a time, parents and doctors can
more easily isolate what vaccine is the culprit if a severe reaction does occur. This helps them decide when and how to repeat reactive vaccines.

If some of the theoretical problems with vaccines are real, this
schedule circumvents most of them. If the problems aren't real,
then the only drawback is the extra time, effort, and cost for the

additional doctor's office visits. It means more gas money, more co-pays, and more "scary" episodes for your child. Oh, and you risk really annoying your doctor because you're trying to think outside the box. However, it does eventually provide complete protection from diseases, and it does so at an age-appropriate pace. It gives kids protection from diseases at the ages when those diseases are the most troublesome, and it doesn't unnecessarily overload young kids with vaccines that they don't really need until they're older.

This schedule would probably drive public health officials crazy. In large cities, where some families don't have good access to health care (whether from lack of insurance, language barriers, or financial reasons), it's already a challenge to get kids fully vaccinated. If we double the number of visits needed, we can forget any goal of achieving high vaccination levels in some areas. Yet ultimately, the choice is yours if you think the precautions are worth it.

I know that this alternative schedule is very different from the one your doctor will want to give your kids. Many doctors will fight you if you try to "change the system." But if you copy this schedule, show it to your doctor, and explain your reasons, you'll show him or her that you have thoroughly thought the issue through. You aren't saying "no" to vaccines, you are just spreading them out. The doctor may see your logic, won't look at you as if you're crazy, and will go along with your choices.

I actually think that this alternative vaccine schedule can *increase* vaccination rates in our country, not *decrease* them. Many parents are choosing not to vaccinate simply because they lack information and they lack options.

But a vaccine schedule that resolves much of the controversy and minimizes the side effects of vaccines can make leery parents feel more confident in the system. So in order to gain more cooperation from the doubters, we doctors need to give a little. We need to meet them halfway. We need to offer them a schedule that acknowledges their concerns but doesn't compromise disease protection.

Whatever vaccine schedule you choose, I hope that you now think you can make a fully educated decision for your children.

Update: In 2009 Merck decided to stop producing the separate measles, mumps, and rubella vaccines. Separating this vaccine is a prominent feature of my alternative vaccine schedule. Unfortunately, that option is no longer available to you. You'll have to decide whether your child should get the full MMR at age 1 and 5 as recommended by the CDC, or whether you should delay it or skip it altogether. My advice is to go ahead and have your child vaccinated as recommended if you feel comfortable doing so. If you have concerns about the MMR, delay it. You could safely delay the vaccine until your child enters school, since he is unlikely to come into contact with anyone who has one of these three illnesses. Once a child enters daycare or school, however, the chance of exposure increases. So I do recommend that a child get the MMR prior to daycare or school entry. Those children who do not receive the vaccine until age 4 only need one dose, as the vaccine works better the older the child is. Those who get the vaccine at age 2 or 3 may or may not need a second dose at age 5. Your doctor can do a blood test at age 5 to determine if the one dose worked well enough before you automatically proceed with the second dose. I would also recommend that the MMR be given several months away from any other vaccine. I will provide further information and updates regarding this issue at www.TheVaccineBook.com.

Afterword

Wow! You made it through. That was a seriously long book. Not like *War and Peace,* but, given the subject matter, it did seem longer than a Russian winter. But wait. You aren't done yet. You still have to read the afterword, and I guarantee it will be worth your time. Most "afterwords" are just an author's way of saying good-bye. Many of us don't want to stop writing, so we just keep rambling on. We don't want the book to end. We think that as long as we don't put the pen down, insightful revelations will continue to flow onto the page. We might as well make it a whole ending chapter instead of tricking people into thinking the book is done. Oops, sorry. Where was I? Oh, yeah. This afterword is nothing of the sort. I promise I'll stop writing when I run out of useful things to say.

Are you wondering how I got so interested in vaccines? Thirteen years ago, my wife and I were trying to relocate to the West Coast after medical school, and we needed a place to live for a month. My wife's friend and her husband offered to let us stay with them, but with one condition. The husband asked me to read a book while we were there. Not just any book—an anti-vaccine book. I figured it was the least I could do for free rent. I didn't believe much of that book at the time, but one thing caught my attention. It cited several medical studies that discussed vaccine side effects. I had always thought there were some theoretical side effects from vaccines, but I'd brushed them off as so rare that they weren't worth thinking about. I went to the library at my medical school and looked up the studies. Sure enough, the book was right. Vaccines do have some well-documented side effects. Some are quite severe but fortunately rare. (Even more interesting is that the very vaccine that our friend's book was written about, the old whole-cell DTP, has since been taken off the market because of its side effects.) This chance reading started me on a very long road of research and discovery, and *The Vaccine Book* is the culmination of my thirteen years of study.

My friend had an ulterior motive. He was very active in the anti-vaccine movement, and having a young and impressionable doctor living under his roof was his chance to influence me. We became close friends over the years as we debated back and forth. As a rocket scientist (he literally builds rockets and satellites for a living), he often seemed to outsmart me. And he did succeed in making me think.

Every single day, parents in my office ask me about vaccinations. They ask me if they are safe and what the side effects are. They ask me if the diseases are common or rare. They want to know more details before their children get the shots. Life was probably so much easier for doctors in the old days when good patients just did whatever the doctor told them without question. I'll never know what that was like because, as a young doctor, I am surrounded by the kinds of parents who like to ask questions and don't follow my advice blindly. Because I used to be one of those annoyingly educated parents when my kids were young, I can empathize. I understand their worries.

Most of the parents I encounter in my office vaccinate their kids. Some choose not to vaccinate, and as long as I make sure they understand the risks of the diseases, I've learned to accept their freedom of choice. I'm surprised, however, that before coming to me, many of these families were actually kicked out of their previous pediatricians' offices over this issue. It seems as if I'm one of the few doctors in the O.C. (that's Orange County, California, for those of you who don't watch TV) who accepts patients who don't vaccinate.

Why are many doctors not open to discussing the pros and cons of vaccines with their patients? One doctor I talked to summed it up perfectly. He is an infectious disease specialist, and he was very honest in telling me he is biased when it comes to shots. That's because he sees all the bad things that can happen when a child is overcome by a vaccine-preventable disease. He sees kids die from chickenpox. He sees kids with brain damage from meningitis. He sees kids who need liver transplants because of hepatitis infections. He sees kids die from complications of the flu. If I lived in his world, I would probably be far more pro-vaccine than I am. All it takes is one very bad case of a disease to convince a doctor that anyone who opposes vaccines is crazy. Fortunately for me (and even more so for my patients!), I almost never see kids suffer complications from vaccine-preventable infectious diseases. Death and disability from disease is a hard thing for any doctor to stomach, so it's no wonder that most are pro-vaccine.

What I really don't understand is why many doctors kick patients out of their practice over this issue. What's wrong with simply disagreeing with parents but still providing medical care to their child? That's what the American Academy of Pediatrics tells us we should do (see page xviii). Read them the riot act once, then move on and be their doctor. A family that chooses not to vaccinate still needs medical care. Sure, their child may catch a vaccine-preventable disease, and yes, their unvaccinated child decreases the local herd immunity and puts other kids at risk, but that is still their choice. Parents of patients refuse to follow my medical advice every day. I can tell a mom to stop buying junk food for her overweight child or she risks obesity-related diseases, but does she listen? I tell a dad he needs to stop smoking or his kids will suffer the consequences of secondhand smoke, but does he stop? I ask a mom to baby-proof her house to keep her toddler from choking, but does she follow my advice? Some do, some don't. Do I kick these patients out of my practice? No. Do I patiently inform them of the risks they're taking with their kid's health? Of course. Then I get over it. I'm there to serve them, not the other way around. Do doctors have the time to inform each and every patient who asks questions about vaccines what all the pros and cons are? That's what books are for. This book in particular.

I admit that one reason I wrote this book is purely a selfish one. Because I was bombarded with vaccine questions every day, I put together a seminar a few years ago that was an abbreviated version of everything you read here. Each month I had about twenty parents sitting in my waiting room for two hours while I went through all these details with them. This way, I didn't have to answer individual questions in the office. I could do it once a month instead.

Well, after four years and forty-eight seminars, it began to get a little old. Not old for my patients, of course, who hungrily ate up every piece of information I gave them, but for me. Each evening seminar was an evening away from my family. I decided I would write it all down so I could stop giving the seminars. Parents in my practice are still going to have some questions, even after reading this book, but they now have a written reference as well.

What do I hope you have gained from this book? If you were already *anti*-vaccine before you began reading, then I hope I've given you some things to think about. I've also given you a better understanding of the diseases so you know what risks you are taking by not vaccinating your child. I have also given you a heads-up on what two states in the country you shouldn't move to if you want to keep your children (see page 218). If you are pretty much *pro*-vaccine and plan to have your child get all the shots, I hope I've given you a good understanding of the possible side effects and some ideas about how to vaccinate as safely as you can. I think spreading out the shots to avoid overloading young babies with aluminum and other chemicals is a very good idea. For the rest of you, who want to partially vaccinate your kids, I've tried to help you understand which shots are most important and how to administer them in the safest way possible.

I do think that vaccines are very important, but I wish more attention were given to safety research and the possible problems with vaccines. Had we paid more attention and had better safeguards, problems like reactions from the old DTP vaccine, thimerosal, and the SV-40 virus in polio vaccines could have been avoided. And I think there's still room for improvement. I wish we could find a way to make vaccines without using animal or human tissues. I wish we could make vaccines without aluminum and other chemicals. I have a dream. In my dream we have the best of both worlds—a world free of harmful infectious diseases and vaccines that are completely 100 percent safe. Can this happen someday? Yes. Will it take a lot of work? You bet. As public awareness of the few problems with vaccines increases, so will the medical and pharmaceutical communities' desire to develop safer vaccines. I want our nation's vaccine schedule to be the safest it possibly can be. I want parents everywhere to feel confident in and comfortable with the vaccines they give their children.

I hope I've answered all your questions. I am honored to have had the privilege to offer you guidance on this confusing and controversial topic. Your children are precious, and you have the right to make informed medical decisions for them. I wish you the best.

Vaccines and Diseases at a Glance

	HIB	**Pc**	**DTaP**	**Hep B**	**Rotavirus**	**Polio**
			VACCINE			
Disease common	N	Y	Pertussis —Yes	N	Y	N
Disease severe	Y	Y	Y	Y	Y	Y
Contains aluminum	Varies by brand	Y	Y	Y	N	N
High chemical content	N	N	Y	Y	N	Y
Uses human or animal tissues	N	N	Varies by brand	N	Y	Y
Long list of side effects	N	N	N	Y	N	N
Higher risk of severe side effects	N	N	N	Y	N	N
World travel a higher risk than in U.S.	Y	N	Diph —Yes	N	N	Y

	MMR	**Chickenpox**	**Hep A**	**Flu**	**Meningo-coccal**	**HPV**
			VACCINE			
Disease common	N	Y	Y	Y	N	Y
Disease severe	N	N	N	Y	Y	Y
Contains aluminum	N	N	Y	N	N	Y
High chemical content	N	N	Y	Y	N	N
Uses human or animal tissues	Y	Y	Y	Y	N	N
Long list of side effects	Y	Y	N	Y	N	N
Higher risk of severe side effects	Y	Y	N	Y	Y	N
World travel a higher risk than in U.S.	Y	N	Y	N	N	N

Resources

I have included a long list of research articles for two reasons. First, sections of this book discuss various problems with vaccines, and it would be irresponsible of me to include these issues without providing the resources that I used to write about them. Second, most doctors—myself included until thirteen years ago—are unaware that there are numerous articles in mainstream medical journals that discuss vaccine side effects and potential problems. I have included a number of these articles, not to suggest that I believe they are all true, but just to point out that many doctors around the world have researched vaccine safety, found some potential problems, and published their findings in mainstream journals. I want you to be able to read them on your own. Still, the vast majority of research published in these same medical journals shows that vaccines are safe and effective. For every article listed that discusses a vaccine side effect, there are several other articles that find there isn't enough evidence to prove that vaccines cause most of the noted reactions. I haven't cited many of those other articles because they are numerous and can easily be found by searching the topics online.

ALUMINUM TOXICITY

Articles stating there are no harmful effects from aluminum in vaccines:

Adverse events after immunization with aluminum-containing DTP vaccines: systematic review of the evidence, Jefferson T. et al., *Lancet: Infectious Diseases* 2004; 4:84–90.

Summary: This report from the Cochrane Group didn't find any evidence that the DTP vaccine caused harmful aluminum-related side effects.

Articles discussing potential problems from aluminum in vaccines:

Aluminum toxicity in infants and children, Committee on Nutrition, American Academy of Pediatrics, *Pediatrics* 1996; 97:413–416.

Summary: This article is discussed in the text. See page 199.

ASPEN statement on aluminum in parenteral nutrition solutions, Charney P., Aluminum Task Force, *Nutrition in Clinical Practice* 2004; 19:416–417.

Summary: This article is discussed in the text. See page 196.

Federal Food, Drug, and Cosmetic Act for dextrose injections, Document NDA 19-626/S-019, Department of Health and Human Services, Food and Drug Administration. Available online at www.fda.gov/cder/foi/appletter/2004/19626scs019ltr.pdf.

Summary: This article is discussed in the text. See page 195.

Aluminum in large and small volume parenterals used in total parenteral nutrition, Document 02N-0496, Department of Health and Human Services, Food and Drug Administration. Available online at www.fda.gov/ohrms/dockets/98fr/oc0367.pdf.

Summary: This article is discussed in the text. See page 196.

Effects of aluminum on the neurotoxicity of primary cultured neurons and on the aggregation of beta-amyloid protein, Kawahara M. et al., *Brain Research Bulletin* 2001; 55:211–217.

Summary: Researchers at the Department of Molecular and Cellular Neurobiology, Tokyo Metropolitan Institute for Neuroscience, Japan, exposed rat nerve cells to varying amounts of aluminum and found not only nerve degeneration but also accumulation of amyloid proteins, as is seen in patients with Alzheimer's disease. The levels of aluminum needed to cause this effect was 50 micromoles over a three-week period. It isn't clear how 50 micromoles compares to microgram units in the vaccines.

Aluminum-adjuvanted vaccines transiently increase aluminum levels in murine brain tissue, Redhead K., Quinlan G. J., Das R. G., Gutteridge J. M., *Pharmacology and Toxicology* 1992; 70:278–280.

Summary: This group from England injected aluminum-containing vaccines into mice and found that levels of the metal rose in the brain and peaked around the third day after injection.

Aluminum impairs the glutamate-nitric oxide-cGMP pathway in cultured neurons and in rat brain in vivo: molecular mechanisms and implications for neuropathology, Canales J. J. et al., *Journal of Inorganic Biochemistry* 2001; 87(1–2):63–69.

Summary: This group from Spain found that when pregnant rats were fed aluminum long-term, the brains of their babies showed impaired biochemistry (as described in the title of the paper).

Effects of aluminum exposure on brain glutamate and GABA systems: an experimental study in rats, Nayak P., Chatterjee A. K., *Food and Chemical Toxicology* 2001; 39(12):1285–1289.

Summary: This group from the University of Calcutta, India, had findings similar to the study above.

Aluminum neurotoxicity in preterm infants receiving intravenous feeding solutions, Bishop N. J., Morley R., Day J. P., Lucas A., *New England Journal of Medicine* 1997; 336(22):1557–1561.

Summary: This Cambridge group found that premature human

infants given standard IV feeding solutions containing aluminum had impaired neurologic and mental development compared to infants fed nonaluminum solutions.

Neuropathology of aluminum toxicity in rats (glutamate and GABA impairment), El-Rhaman S. S., *Pharmacological Research* 2003; 47(3): 189–194.

Summary: This group fed aluminum to rats for thirty-five days and found high levels of the metal in the brain tissue, as well as brain tissue degeneration in a pattern similar to that of Alzheimer's disease.

VACCINES AND CHRONIC DISEASES

Studies showing that some chronic diseases may be triggered by vaccines:

Unexplained fever in neonates may be associated with hepatitis B vaccine, Linder N. et al., *Archives of Disease in Childhood: Fetal and Neonatal Edition* 1999; 81(3):206–207.

Summary: This group compared five thousand infants born at their medical center in 1991, before hep B vaccination began, to the five thousand born in 1992 who were given the vaccine at birth. Fourteen unvaccinated infants were admitted with fever in the first three days of life in the 1991 unvaccinated group, and thirty-five infants were admitted for fever in the 1992 vaccinated group. They concluded that there may be some infants who unnecessarily undergo testing and treatment for fevers due to the vaccine and that further research should be done.

The first central nervous system demyelinization and hepatitis B vaccination: a pilot case control study, Touze E. et al., *Revue Neurologique* (Paris) 2000; 156(3):242–246.

Summary: This French group studied 240 cases of CNS demyelination (similar to Guillain-Barré syndrome, see page 181) that occurred in

1993 through 1995. After determining any timely relationship to getting a hep B vaccine, they concluded that they could not exclude the possibility that hep B vaccine may have been associated with these events.

Rheumatic disorders developed after hepatitis B vaccination, Maillefert J. F. et al., *Rheumatology* 1999; 38(10):978–983.

Summary: This group reported on twenty-two cases of inflammatory or autoimmune diseases following hep B vaccine in France, including six cases of rheumatoid arthritis and two cases of lupus.

Acute sero-positive rheumatoid arthritis occurring after hepatitis vaccination, Vautier G., Carty J. E., *British Journal of Rheumatology* 1994; 33:991.
Reactive arthritis after hepatitis B vaccination, Hachulla E. et al., *Journal of Rheumatology* 1990; 179:1250–1251.
Thrombocytopenia purpura after recombinant hepatitis B vaccine, Poullin P., Gabriel B., *Lancet* 1994; 344:1293.

Summary: These three papers discuss specific cases of the noted observed reactions in patients who received hep B vaccine.

Vaccinations and multiple sclerosis, Gout O., Federation of Neurology, Paris, *Neurological Science* 2001; 22(2):151–154.

Summary: This paper discusses the several hundred reports of MS-like reactions after hep B vaccine during the 1990s. They could find no actual proof that the vaccine was related. They discuss possible theories of how the vaccine may trigger this reaction.

Arthritis after hepatitis B vaccination: report of three cases, Gross K. et al., *Scandinavian Journal of Rheumatology* 1995; 24(1):50–52.

Summary: This article reports on three cases of severe arthritis after hep B vaccination. One patient developed rheumatoid arthritis (a lifelong autoimmune arthritis).

Atopic dermatitis is increased following vaccination for measles, mumps, and rubella or measles infection, Olesen A. B. et al., *Acta Dermato-venereologica* 2003; 83(6):445–450.

Summary: These researchers found that atopic dermatitis (eczema) was more common after kids get the MMR vaccine or catch a natural measles infection. They discuss how early exposure to infections can affect the immune system and trigger eczema. They suggest that further research be done on this issue.

Clustering of cases of insulin dependent diabetes (IDDM) occurring three years after hemophilus influenza B (HiB) immunization support causal relationship between immunization and IDDM, Classen J. B., Classen D. C., *Autoimmunity* 2003; 36(3):123.

Summary: This study looked at 116,000 kids who got the HIB vaccine in Finland during its first two years of use. They found that child-onset diabetes was significantly more common in those kids compared to 128,000 kids who were born two years earlier and did not receive the vaccine. They also found that the vaccine triggered diabetes in mice.

Vaccination-induced cutaneous pseudolymphoma, Maubec E. et al., *Journal of the American Academy of Dermatology* 2005; 52(4):623–629.

Summary: This is a report on nine patients who developed pseudolymphoma on the skin where they'd been given an aluminum-containing vaccine (hep B or hep A). Pseudolymphoma is an inflammatory condition on the skin in which lymphoid tissue overgrows and resembles lymphoma. Aluminum deposits were also found.

Vaccine-induced autoimmunity, Cohen A. D., *Journal of Autoimmunity* 1996; 9(6):699–703.

Summary: This paper reviews reports of autoimmune disorders after vaccination, discusses the possible mechanisms that are occurring, and suggests that further research be done. It also states that the benefits of vaccines outweigh these risks.

Kawasaki disease in an infant following immunization with hepatitis B vaccine, Miron D., *Clinical Rheumatology* 2003; 22(6):461–463.

Summary: This article concerns a one-month-old baby who developed Kawasaki disease (a life-threatening inflammation of the heart and blood vessels) one day after the second hep B dose. It also mentions that similar vasculitic reactions have been reported in adults getting the hep B vaccine.

Vaccination and autoimmunity "vaccinosis": a dangerous liaison? Shoenfeld Y., Aron-Maor A., *Journal of Autoimmunity* 2000; 14(1):1–10.

Summary: This discussion paper acknowledges that many autoimmune reactions have been reported after vaccines. The authors state that in many cases vaccines can't be proved to be responsible but that there's enough evidence to suggest a relationship. They point out that the timing of the reactions (often two to three months after vaccination) is very consistent with autoimmune reactions.

Macrophagic myofasciitis lesions assess long-term persistence of vaccine-derived aluminum hydroxide in muscle, Gherardi M. et al., *Brain* 2001; 124(9):1821–1831.

Summary: This group at the University of Paris studied fifty cases of this condition (which causes severe muscle and joint pain and fatigue) and found that all had aluminum-induced muscle inflammation at the site of an aluminum-containing vaccine injection as long as three years prior.

Note: Numerous studies have also been published that show there's not enough evidence to prove a link between these vaccines and the chronic diseases mentioned above. I have not included them here because they are too numerous to list.

MMR VACCINE AND AUTISM

Studies showing no link between MMR vaccine and autism or other neurodevelopmental disorders:

Vaccines for measles, mumps, and rubella in children, *The Cochrane Database of Systematic Reviews* 2005; issue 4.

Summary: This reviews thirty-one research studies on the MMR vaccine. They concluded there was no credible link between MMR vaccine and autism.

No evidence for links between autism, MMR, and measles virus, Chen W. et al., *Psychological Medicine* 2004; 34(3):543–553.

Summary: This study out of London found no evidence that the MMR vaccine, the separate measles vaccine, or natural measles infection were linked to autism. The study did find some rare complications of MMR vaccine.

Immunization Safety Review: Vaccines and Autism, Immunization Safety Review Committee, Washington, DC: Institute of Medicine of the National Academies, 2004.

Summary: This isn't actually a research study. It is a review, summary, and consensus opinion of available research. They conclude that there is no evidence of a link between vaccines and autism. For more information, go to www.iom.edu.

MMR vaccine and autism: an update of the scientific evidence, DeStefano F., Thompson W. W., Centers for Disease Control, *Expert Review of Vaccines* 2004; 3(1):19–22.

Summary: This isn't a research study. It is a review and summary of other research studies. The authors conclude that the MMR vaccine does not cause autism or gastrointestinal disease.

Epidemiology and possible causes of autism, Hershel J., Kaye J. A., *Pharmacotherapy* 2003; 23(12):1524–1530.

Summary: This group reviewed other research studies involving autism and found that the increased incidence of autism is due to better diagnostic techniques and awareness. They found no evidence linking autism to vaccines.

Unintended events following immunization with MMR: a systematic review, Jefferson T. et al., *Vaccine* 2003; 21(25–26):3954–3960.

Summary: This group reviewed twenty-two studies of the MMR vaccine and concluded that it was unlikely to be associated with autism and various other reported side effects. They did also conclude, however, that "the design and reporting of safety outcomes in MMR vaccine studies, both pre- and post-marketing, are largely inadequate."

A case-control study of measles vaccination and inflammatory bowel disease, The East Dorset Gastroenterology Group, Feeney M. et al., *Lancet* 1997; 350(9080):764–766.

Summary: This group compared the measles vaccination rates of 440 inflammatory bowel disease patients and found that just as many had been vaccinated for measles as not. They concluded that their findings do not support a hypothesis of a link between inflammatory bowel disease and measles vaccine.

Studies showing a possible link between MMR vaccine and autism:

Ileal-lymphoid-nodular hyperplasia, non-specific colitis, and pervasive developmental disorder in children, Wakefield A. et al., *Lancet* 1998; 351:637–641.

Summary: This is the landmark study that began the whole debate. Wakefield found twelve children who developed regressive autism during the second year of life (after the MMR vaccine was given) who also had intestinal inflammatory disease consistent with a viral infection, possibly measles related. See page 94 for further discussion.

Potential viral pathogenic mechanism for new variant inflammatory bowel disease, Uhlmann V. et al, *Molecular Pathology* 2002; 55(2): 84–90.

Summary: This eleven-doctor group in Ireland did intestinal biopsies on a large group of children with autism and found that of the ninety-one kids who showed ileal lymphonodular hyperplasia and enterocolitis, seventy-five had confirmed measles virus infecting their intestinal linings. Only five of the seventy healthy control patients tested showed the measles virus. This study offers more support for Dr. Wakefield's claim of a link between measles virus, inflammatory bowel disease, and autism.

Is measles vaccination a risk factor for inflammatory bowel disease? Thompson N. P. et al., *Lancet* 1995; 345(8957):1071–1074.

Summary: This group of doctors studied thirty-five hundred adult patients with inflammatory bowel disease and other chronic intestinal conditions who had received the measles vaccine in 1964 as part of the vaccine safety trials. When compared to a control group of eleven thousand adults who didn't get the measles vaccine, the vaccinated people were three times more likely to develop inflammatory bowel disease. This study predates Dr. Wakefield's work and is consistent with his concern about a link between the measles vaccine and inflammatory bowel disease.

An investigation of the association between MMR vaccination and autism in Denmark, Goldman G. S., Yazbak F. E., *Journal of American Physicians and Surgeons* 2004; 9(3):70–75.

Summary: This group studied the incidence of autism in Denmark before the MMR vaccine was introduced compared to its incidence in the years thereafter. They found about a 400 percent increase in autism over those years. This group used the same data as the two Denmark studies listed on page 259, which concluded that there is not enough evidence to link mercury in vaccines to autism. In this study, however, Goldman's group concluded that there may be a link between the MMR vaccine and autism in Denmark.

Detection of measles virus genomic RNA in cerebrospinal fluid of children with regressive autism: a report of three cases, Bradstreet J. J. et al., *Journal of American Physicians and Surgeons* 2004; 9(2):38–45.

Summary: This group found measles virus RNA in the CSF and intestinal biopsies of three children who had gastrointestinal inflammatory disease and autism. The only known exposure these kids ever had was from the MMR vaccine. Three control patients did not have measles detected in their samples.

Gastrointestinal symptoms and intestinal disaccharidase activities in children with autism, Kushak R. et al., *Journal of Pediatric Gastroenterology and Nutrition* 2005; 41(4):508.

Summary: This Harvard group essentially reproduced Dr. Andrew Wakefield's work by finding chronic inflammation, lymphoid hyperplasia, and digestive enzyme deficiency in the gastrointestinal tract of numerous autistic children. It didn't explore a possible link to measles infection from the MMR vaccine, however.

A comparative evaluation of the effects of MMR immunization and mercury doses from thimerosal-containing childhood vaccines on the population prevalence of autism, Geier D. A., Geier M. R., *Medical Science Monitor* 2004; 10(3):PI33–139.

Summary: This group studied the increase in autism over the past twenty years compared with the timing of increased thimerosal vaccines and the introduction of the MMR vaccine and found evidence that these may play a role in neurodevelopmental disorders. They recommended taking thimerosal out of vaccines and finding a safer MMR vaccine.

Studies showing no link between mercury (thimerosal) in vaccines and autism:

Thimerosal and the occurence of autism: negative ecological evidence from Danish population-based data, Madsen K. M., *Pediatrics* 2003; 112(3 Pt 1):604–606.

Summary: This study showed that the incidence of autism in Denmark continued to increase after thimerosal was removed from vaccines. It concluded that thimerosal is not linked to autism.

Autism and thimerosal-containing vaccines: lack of consistent evidence for an association, Stehr-Green P., *American Journal of Preventive Medicine* 2003; 25(2):101–106.

Summary: This group compared the rates of autism in California, Sweden, and Denmark with the introduction and removal of thimerosal-containing vaccines. While the study did show an increase in autism with the increase of thimerosal vaccines, they did *not* see a decrease in autism when thimerosal was removed from vaccines in Sweden and Denmark. They therefore concluded that there is not enough evidence to suggest a link.

Studies showing a possible link between mercury (thimerosal) in vaccines and autism:

"1991 Memo Warned of Mercury in Shots," Levin M., *Los Angeles Times*, February 8, 2005.
    Summary: This article is discussed in the text. See page 206.

Early downward trends in neurodevelopmental disorders following removal of thimerosal-containing vaccines, Geier D. A., Geier M. R., *Journal of American Physicians and Surgeons* 2006; 11(1):8–13.
    Summary: This study, similar to the other Geier study on page 259, found not only that autism increased in the United States as the number of thimerosal-containing vaccines increased but also that autism has begun to decrease since thimerosal was removed from U.S. vaccines in 2002.

Mercury and autism: accelerating evidence? Mutter J. et al., *Neuroendocrinology Letters* 2005; 26(5):439–446.
    Summary: This laboratory study found that vaccine concentrations of thimerosal inhibit a brain enzyme (methionine synthetase) necessary for neurologic function and detoxification. They note that autistic kids also show this same enzyme dysfunction.

Neurotoxic effects of postnatal thimerosal are mouse strain dependent, Hornig M. et al., *Molecular Psychiatry* 2004; 9:833–845.
    Summary: These researchers gave a group of mice injections of thimerosal at two, four, six, and twelve months of age (an amount equivalent by weight to what a human infant would have received from vaccines). They found that the mice suffered neurologic and behavior effects similar to those seen in autism.

Porphyrinuria in childhood autistic disorder: implications for environmental toxicity, Nataf R. et al., *Toxicology and Applied Pharmacology* 2006; 214(2):99–108.
    Summary: This study looked at urine levels of a compound called porphyrin (which is elevated in people with heavy metal-poisoning) in

269 kids with neurodevelopmental disorders, including autism. They found that the levels were elevated in autistic kids. The levels decreased after undergoing metal detoxification treatment with DMSA.

VACCINE SIDE EFFECTS

Information on side effects of separate measles and mumps vaccine:

Neurologic disorders following live measles-virus vaccination, Landrigan P., Witte J., *Journal of the American Medical Association* 1973; 223(13):1459–1462.

Summary: This is a report on fifty-nine cases of encephalitis or encephalopathy and one case of subacute sclerosing panencephalitis (see page 182) occurring six to fifteen days after vaccination with live measles vaccine in the United States between 1963 and 1971. During that time, about fifty million doses had been distributed. They therefore calculated the risk of a severe neurologic reaction to be about one in a million.

Mumps meningitis following MMR immunization, Gray J., Burns S., *Lancet* 1989; 2(8654):98.

Summary: This is a case report of a child with mumps meningitis following vaccination. The virus was later identified as the vaccine strain, not natural mumps; *Lancet* 1989; 2(8668):927.

Mumps meningitis, possibly vaccine related, Azzopardi P., *Ontario Canada Disease Weekly Report* 1988; 14:209–210.

Summary: This is a report on three cases of this occurrence in Canada.

Mumps meningitis following MMR immunization, Muhlendahl K., *Lancet* 1989; 2:394.

Summary: This is a report of one case of this occurrence and a reminder about eight other cases from Canada.

Mumps vaccine and meningitis, Ehrengut W., *Lancet* 1989; 2(8665):751.

Summary: This is a report on eight cases of mumps meningitis and four cases of encephalitis or encephalopathy following mumps vaccine that occurred in Germany.

Note: Researchers feel these cases of mumps meningitis occurred because the virus wasn't weakened enough during the manufacturing process. The newer MMR vaccine used today is made with a slightly different process and may not cause as many cases as the older vaccines did.

Information on side effects of rubella vaccines:

Adverse events following pertussis and rubella vaccines, Howson C., Fineberg H., The Institute of Medicine, *Journal of the American Medical Association* 1992; 267(3):392–396.

Summary: This group reviewed many research studies and found that the rubella vaccine *can* cause acute arthritis (15 percent chance) and *may* cause chronic arthritis (they were unable to estimate an actual percent chance of this) in adult women. Arthritis was much less common in children, teens, and male adults.

Arthritis associated with induced rubella infection, Ogra P., Herd K., *The Journal of Immunology* 1971; 107(3):810–813.

Summary: This study discusses the cases of four children who suffered severe prolonged arthritis after a rubella vaccine.

Persistent rubella infection and rubella-associated arthritis, Chantler J. et al., *Lancet* 1982; 1(8285):1323–1325.

Summary: This is a report on six women who developed chronic arthritis for up to six years following rubella vaccination (an older form of the vaccine, not the one used today).

Is RA27/3 rubella immunization a cause of chronic fatigue? Allen A., *Medical Hypotheses* 1998; 27:217–220.

Summary: This paper discusses the finding that many women with chronic fatigue syndrome have rubella antibody levels much higher than average and that chronic fatigue syndrome surfaced in the literature three years after the new rubella vaccine was developed.

Information on the possibility that HIB vaccine may temporarily increase a baby's susceptibility to catching HIB disease:

Hemophilus influenzae type B disease in children vaccinated with type B polysaccharide vaccine, Granoff D. et al., *The New England Journal of Medicine* 1986; 315:1584–1590.

Summary: This is a report of fifty-five cases of HIB meningitis that occurred three or more weeks after immunization with HIB vaccine. These kids were found to have an extremely low antibody response to the disease compared to twenty-five patients who had HIB meningitis and had never been vaccinated (their antibody response was six times higher than the vaccinated kids'). Somehow the vaccine seemed to prevent these kids' immune systems from responding to the natural disease.

Decline in serum antibody to the capsule of *Haemophilus influenzae* type B in the immediate postimmunization period, Daum R. et al., *The Journal of Pediatrics* 1989; 114(5): 742–747.

Summary: Thirty-two infants and sixteen adults were given the HIB vaccine and their antibody levels were monitored for the next five days. All of the adults and most of the infants showed a significant decrease in HIB antibodies that lasted about five days. The researchers concluded that this might increase the risk of severe HIB disease if someone is exposed to the germ right before or after vaccination.

Postvaccination susceptibility to invasive *Haemophilus influenzae* type b disease in infant rats, Sood S. et al., *The Journal of Pediatrics* 1988; 113(5):814–819.

Summary: This group immunized rats against HIB, then injected them with HIB bacteria. Most of the vaccinated rats caught severe HIB disease, whereas only some of the unvaccinated control group caught HIB when injected.

INCIDENCE OF HEPATITIS B IN CHILDREN

The changing epidemiology of hepatitis B in the United States. Need for alternative vaccination strategies, Alter M. J., Hadler S. C., Margolis H. S., et al., *Journal of the American Medical Association* 1990; 263: 1218–1222.

Summary: This group found that about one-third of people who catch hep B did not have any identifiable risk factors (sex with multiple partners, IV drug use, etc.). They recommended that all infants be immunized to decrease the incidence of hep B transmission in low-risk populations. One of the authors of this study went on to work for a hep B vaccine manufacturer (Beecham Labs, which later merged with SmithKline), according to a footnote on the first page of the paper.

Prevention of hepatitis B virus infection in the United States: a pediatric perspective, West D. J., Margolis H. S., *Pediatric Infectious Disease Journal* 1992; 11:866–874.

Summary: This paper summarizes the results from numerous research studies that suggested that hep B is much more common than the actual number of reported cases. They estimated that two hundred thousand new cases of hep B occur each year in the United States. Merck Laboratories, a maker of hep B vaccine, is listed as the sponsor of this paper, and one of these doctors worked for Merck, according to a footnote on the first page of the paper.

Hepatitis B: evolving epidemiology and implications for control, Margolis H.S., Alter M. J., Hadler S. C., *Seminars in Liver Disease* 1991; 11(2):84–92.

Summary: These researchers used statistical analysis and epidemiological studies to estimate that as many as 30,000 infants and children must be getting infected with hep B every year in ways other than exposure at birth. This finding was a driving force in hep B vaccine becoming routine for all infants.

Estimated and reported cases of hepatitis B infection in children, Sepkowitz S., *Pediatric Infectious Disease Journal* 1993; 12(6):542–544.

Summary: This is a letter from a doctor who raised numerous questions about Dr. Margolis's conclusions, stating that his estimates are too high and that the actual number of infant hep B cases is very low. Dr. Margolis's response letter is provided on the same page.

Achievements in public health: hepatitis B vaccination, United States, 1982 to 2002, *Morbidity and Mortality Weekly Report* 2002; 51(25):549–552, 563. Available online at www.cdc.gov/mmwr/preview/mmwrhtml/mm5125a3.htm.

Summary: This is the paper where I found the actual number of reported childhood cases of hep B infection to be very low, only 360 per year (as opposed to the overly estimated 30,000 cases that were thought to be occurring). This number comes from the chart at the end of the paper, which states that in the late 1980s and early 1990s there was about 1 case for every 100,000 kids each year in our population of kids ages 0 through 9 years. According to the U.S. Census Bureau, there were about 36,000,000 kids in that age group in 1990. This means there were about 360 cases reported in children ages 0 through 9 each year. See page 51 for this discussion.

PROBLEMS WITH THE OLD DTP VACCINE

An evaluation of serious neurological disorders following immunization: a comparison of whole-cell pertussis and acellular pertussis vaccines, Geier D. A., Geier M. R., *Brain and Development* 2004; 26(5):296–300.

Summary: This study highlights the significant number of reports of serious neurological side effects from the old DTP vaccine and the comparatively few such reports from the new DTaP vaccine.

Diphtheria-tetanus-pertussis immunization and sudden infant death syndrome, Walker A. M. et al., *American Journal of Public Health* 1987; 77(8):945–951.

Summary: This group studied the cases of SIDS in the United States and found that SIDS occurred seven times more often within three days following DTP vaccine compared to the number of SIDS cases that occurred more than thirty days after vaccination. They concluded that although the SIDS mortality ratio after DTP vaccine was high, the period of risk was relatively short.

Adverse events following pertussis and rubella vaccines, Howson C. P., Fineberg H. V., The Institute of Medicine, *Journal of the American Medical Association* 1992; 267(3):392–396.

Summary: This group reviewed numerous research studies and concluded that the DTP vaccine (the old whole-cell one) *can* cause extended periods of inconsolable screaming (0.1 percent to 6 percent chance) and *may* cause encephalopathy (as high as a 1 in 100,000 chance) and shock (risk ranges from 1 in 30,000 to 1 in 300 chance).

Sudden infant death and immunization: an extensive epidemiological approach to the problem in France, Bouvier-Colle M. H. et al., *International Journal of Epidemiology* 1989; 18(1):121–126.

Summary: This group studied five cases of SIDS following DTP and polio vaccine, compared these to other cases of SIDS, and found no evidence that the vaccines were related.

Pertussis vaccine and injury to the brain, Golden G. S., *Journal of Pediatrics* 1991; 118(3):491–492.

Summary: This study reviewed available literature over the past decades and found no evidence to support a relationship between DTP vaccine and neurologic problems.

Note: There were dozens of studies during the 1980s that looked at the side effects of DTP vaccine and its possible relationship to SIDS or neurologic damage. Some studies found a possible link; some didn't. Because this vaccine is no longer used, it's not anything you really need to think about anyway. I just put these resources here to back up my statement regarding SIDS on page 182.

INCIDENCE AND FATALITY RATES OF PERTUSSIS DISEASE

Pertussis—United States, 2001–2003, Centers for Disease Control, *Morbidity and Mortality Weekly Report* 2005; 54(50):1283–1286.

Summary: You can find this article by going to www.cdc.gov and clicking on *MMWR* under publications, then searching pertussis. I include this as a resource because the data on pertussis fatality rates were fairly hard for me to track down.

INCIDENCE OF FLU IN INFANTS

Trends in pneumonia and influenza morbidity and mortality, American Lung Association, Research and Scientific Affairs Epidemiology and Statistics Unit, August 2004. Available online at www.lungusa.org/atf/cf%7B7A8D42C2-FCCA-4604-8ADE-7F5D5E762256%7D/PI1.PDF.

Summary: This article is discussed in the text. See page 122.

Influenza-associated deaths among children in the United States, 2003–2004, Influenza Special Investigations Team, Bhat N. et al., *New England Journal of Medicine* 2005; 353:2559–2567.

Summary: This team found only 153 reported deaths from the flu in kids seventeen years and younger in one year.

STATE VACCINATION LAWS

Johns Hopkins Institute for Vaccine Safety, www.vaccinesafety.edu.

Summary: Article on state vaccination requirements.

UPDATED VACCINE PRODUCT INSERTS

Updated vaccine product inserts are available at http://users.adelphia.net/~cdc/Vaccines.htm.

MSG

Excitotoxins: The Taste That Kills, Blaylock R. L., Santa Fe, NM: Health Press, 1997.

Summary: This book cites research published in the *Journal of Children's Neurology* 1989; 4:218–226, *Neurosciences Research Program Bulletin* 1981; 19, and *Advances in Neurology: Alzheimer's Disease* 1990; 51, that shows MSG can damage brain cells (see page 209) when consumed in large quantities (several thousand milligrams). The amount in vaccines is only ½ milligram.

SIDE EFFECTS OF PREVNAR VACCINE

Postlicensure safety surveillance for 7-valent pneumococcal conjugate vaccine, Wise R., *Journal of the American Medical Association* 2004; 292:1702–1710.

Summary: This study is discussed on page 18.

INFORMATION ON PNEUMOCOCCAL DISEASE

Impact of the pneumococcal conjugate vaccine on serotype distribution and antimicrobial resistance of invasive *Streptococcus pneumoniae* isolates in Dallas, TX, children from 1999 through 2005, Messina A. et al., *Pediatric Infectious Disease Journal* 2007; 26:461–467.

Summary: This study is discussed on page 18.

MONKEY VIRUS CONTAMINATION OF VACCINES

Case-control study of cancer among U.S. army veterans exposed to simian virus 40–contaminated adenovirus vaccine, Engels E. et al., *American Journal of Epidemiology* 2004; 160:317–324.

Summary: This study is discussed on page 192.

Index